- Malignant diseases

- Steatosis of the liver

- Biliary stone disease

- Arthrosis

- Respiratory problems such as sleep apnea (stopping breathing for short episodes during sleep) and asthma.

- Hormonal imbalance

- Problems with pregnancy and fetal wear

- And others.

And while in older people we can assume that some of the reasons for this are busy everyday life, stress, lack of time to prepare quality food and immobilization, obesity in children is primarily the responsibility of the adults around them. If a child suffers from obesity during childhood and adolescence, the probability of having overweight associated with serious health problems such as an adult increases by between 30% and 60%.

Accordingly, science and health professionals are increasingly beginning to work in the field of early prevention. How can we identify potential health risks, including the risk of obesity, as early as possible, and prevent it, in order to eliminate as far as possible the possibility of developing the disease? Such an approach not only helps to increase people's longevity but also greatly improves its quality.

Customized diet is of great importance. The human diet is strictly personal and varies in different periods of one human life. The child needs a different diet from the adolescent, and a sportsman in order to be healthy and successful in his sport is eating differently from a person who spends most of his time immobile. Therefore, the diet - or else the nutritional regime that we observe at some point in time - must always be personalized to our state and everyday life if we want to help us achieve our goals.

Popular diets do not help this end. With diet, we can lose weight, and if it's curative - to help with our health, but it's only for a certain amount of time. As soon as we return to a typical living environment before diet, usually lost weight and health is back to its former state. In some popular diets, permanent damage to health is observed due to their imbalance and aggression. We do not claim that such diets are ineffective to lose weight - often the followers really manage to significantly reduce their weight. Here the problem is rather the great health risk that accompanies such abrupt weaknesses and often the subsequent weight gain from pre-dieting. It is advisable to reduce the weight by 2-5 kg on average monthly, with adequate nutrition to all individual features - heredity, momentary health status, gender and age, peculiarities of life.

Only lasting, gradual change can help achieve lasting results not only to save health, but also to create the necessary conditions for its improvement. Obesity is a serious condition that needs to be systematically, multilaterally and consistently targeted.

The factors that cause obesity are usually related to the environment in which we live, our way of life, the quantity and quality of our food, and our physical activity, but not only.

But notwithstanding the fact that we are all exposed to the same environment, not everyone develops obesity. It is known that the difference in results obtained in people who follow the same strategies with exercise and diet can often be very large. There is already substantial evidence that such differences are largely regulated by our genes.

In a nutshell, genetics determine the individual's sensitivity to obesity when exposed to an unfavorable environment, and the way he responds to diet and exercise. By rough estimation, genetic factors account for 40% to 80% of body weight differences.

Treat obesity to prevent subsequent complications!

For 2 billion and 500 million years, man acquires his modern appearance by turning the monkey into Homo sapiens. But only in the last few decades has become

Homo obesis - a fat man. The problem is massive and is valid for the whole world, with an emphasis on the most advanced industrial countries. According to WHO estimates, people with obesity are 1 billion and 500 million people. These include overweight and obese obesity. The boundary between normal body weight, overweight and obesity is determined by the so-called BMI - Body Mass Index. It is calculated by dividing the weight in kilograms by the height in meters per square. For normal body weight, BMI is between 18.5 and 24.99, overweight we have an index of 29.99, and obesity - more than 30. According to statistics, a higher percentage of obese are women, secondly, men, but the worst trend is that there are over 43 million children under the age of 5 who are obese. The prospect of them is very bad because they have a very high risk of early development of chronic and potentially debilitating diseases.

What are the causes of the obesity epidemic?

First of all, practically unlimited access and use of high calorie food. Second is the limited physical activity of modern man. When there is a lot of calories in the body, but it is consumed a little, the surplus accumulates in the form of fat. It is a natural process of "stocking" for a period when there will be no food, but it does not happen in our time.

Everyone can compare the everyday life of one person today and 70 to 80 years ago. In the past, almost all activities required physical effort - from moving, through food provision, heating, home maintenance. Today, billions of people are sitting in front of a computer, moving around with cars, escalators and elevators, washing machines and washing dishes, and leisure often goes to bed in front of the TV.

The degree of education and the level of intelligence directly affect the risk of obesity. People who read are more interested in their health, rarely admit overweight, and if they are, for some reason, fathered, more actively and successfully struggling with this problem. Conversely, the low-educated, socially disadvantaged groups are more likely to become obese and do not usually realize that it is a disease that endangers quality and life expectancy.

Contaminated environments, noise, stress also have a bearing on mass obesity.

What is the effect of obesity on health?

According to all scientific studies, overweight and obesity are more common diabetes mellitus, hypertension, ischemic heart disease, including heart attacks, cerebrovascular disease, including strokes, gout, arthrosis in the motor.

According to WHO data, in 2010, 3 million and 400,000 people with obesity died prematurely from various diseases related to excessive weight.

Can weight loss be successfully?

It is entirely possible, but it requires at least two participants - the overweight person and an experienced specialist who can thoroughly assess what measures are needed.

In medical science, it has been shown that overweight reduction is often sufficient to normalize elevated blood pressure, increased blood sugar, high cholesterol. A significant proportion of patients taking medications against hypertension, dyslipidemia, diabetes manage to reduce their dosages and even stop some medications when they normalize their weight.

But one of the serious problems is that a very small part of the overweight and obese people are diagnosed with this disease. The patients themselves tend to perceive their condition as an aesthetic problem rather than a serious illness. And they do not look for any help, even less professional.

Very often obese people make sporadic and chaotic attempts to lose weight and then not only restore high weight but also increase it by entering the so-called "yo-yo" effect. Even more harmful to health is the adoption of various "miraculous" herbs and tablets against overweight.

This problem should be addressed by physicians, especially qualified. Any overweight patient should be thoroughly examined for endocrine causes of high weight. If there is, they are being treated. Then combine hypokaloid diet and physical effort. But on a very well-considered scheme. And when that turns out to be insufficient, there are already proven prescription medications prescribed by a doctor to reduce weight.

Which foods do we need to restrict to get into shape?

There is nothing to exclude, but most people sharply reduce carbohydrates - this behavior usually works. It is desirable to limit the intake of bread, pasta, rice, potatoes, but also to many fruits. They contain sugars that can also have an adverse effect. Sugar beverages as well as alcohol need to be avoided, as well as salt and fat. Nutritionists are for this - to develop independent eating regimes.

With food, can we fight the spring fatigue?

We need to know that food can give, but also take energy from the body. We need a very light dinner to sleep well, otherwise the body works all night and does not rest. Drink at least 2 litres water during the day, eat 2-3 servings of green salad, a little lean meat. For breakfast, take an egg with half a cucumber or a glass of juice. At noon - a salad, spring vegetable soup of spinach, nettles. The light dinner - leafy meals, fish with vegetables - will give us the strength to get fresh and relaxed in the morning.

Should we have breakfast or not?

Breakfast is very important, because with it you provide the necessary energy and nutrients to the next intake. And from the bed, our body constantly moves, its activity starts to rise precisely from the morning hours, as long as its peak at noon and decreases in the afternoon. It is categorical that more frequent eating has a better effect on the whole body, because if we sit down at the table less often, we eat bigger quantities. Accordingly, the liver and kidney function is burdened, blood sugar will fall - that force us to consume more dishes. Last but not least, eating more often improves the energy balance of the body and increases metabolism, and this is one of the keyboards that provide good body weight.

For all these reasons, it is good to have breakfast, and when? It is advisable to be an hour or two after a person wakes up, said the doctors. They advise people, whether they are healthy or have any problems, after getting up to drink a glass of water (if the individual is 60-70 kg) that has body temperature. If a person is bigger (over 90-100 kg), he can drink two glasses. "And I do it every morning because it has a good influence on the gastrointestinal tract, the mucus and waste products released during the night, our body prepares for the upcoming day. After this "ritual", a person who has no problem with weight and is healthy can later drink a fresh juice. For example, carrots, apples, oranges or grapefruit. The choice will be made on the basis of the individual's response - if he has any gastroenterological complaints, the orange or grapefruit is not appropriate, but not if he bets on other fruits, said the nutritionists.

If a person is healthy, they can afford a hearty breakfast (one that includes more complex carbohydrates): with dairy or meat products combined with whole grain bread, another option is sour or fresh milk with cereals. The first meal should be about 300-400 grams or 20-25% of the total amount of the day. And if lunch is not possible, breakfast may be more solid.

If we have to describe what is the first meal for a patient with a disease - for example, overweight, with diabetes and impaired metabolism or with liver or kidney disease, then he should consult a specialist. The doctor will prepare the appropriate menu for him. "However, all these groups of people can brace for breakfast with low-fat dairy or meat products, eat non-fat sour or fresh milk, muesli and oat bran are also a good choice.

It is very important that children are not left without the first meal of the day! It is imperative that they be educated that they should eat regularly and have motor activity, and that means proper growth, development and less gastrointestinal problems.

For breakfast, children must take milk, whether fresh or sour. It is also good if you eat cheese or a local product, but why not an egg, "said the doctor.

What kind of lunch? It has to be the most abundant diet and it is about 35-40% of the daily consumption. "It's good to start with a salad, and if you have gastrointestinal problems and it does not tolerate it, then you can soup, and for the second you can stop lean meals such as vegetables or green beans. You can get meat, chicken, fish, veal, pork (but boiled or roasted), it can be combined with stewed or roasted vegetables. It is good to have a second meal up to 500-700 grams. As for the fruits, eat them between meals. This will ensure gastrointestinal comfort.

Every lady will immediately ask, "When can we afford a dessert and who has fewer calories?" If a person has no problem with the bed or there are no exchange diseases, then he can eat caramel cream, another cream or sour cream. It is good to be light, with less fat and sugar will be degraded and faster), as lunch, as we have said, is the most abundant meal. Some people who asked to eat two soups with a slice of bread at lunch, and yes. "Yes, a vegetable soup of broccoli or tomato with mozzarella with black or whole grain bread is going on," said the specialists.

Dinner should be at 7 pm. at the latest because after 8 pm. the metabolism is shrinking. The body is preparing for sleep. "I recommend a salad with fish or lean meat, maybe stewed vegetables, and the amount of dinner is up to 20-25% of the daily amount of food.

Chocolate? Between meals!?

People who cannot get out of the table without sweetening can eat chocolate, ice cream or fruit milk, but between main meals. And never in the evening - that's very important, experts warn.

And if you're going to get stuck, forget the tempting sweets, pastries and bakery products made from white flour, white rice, and more.

Mediterranean diet

Although it is known as the "diet", the Mediterranean diet is not a diet, but a diet that could be described as a rational diet. It includes consumption of olive oil, fruits, vegetables, cereals, walnuts, fish and red wine, but limits the intake of meat, dairy products and hard alcohol. Strict adherence to the Mediterranean diet is associated with a significantly lower risk of death due to cardiovascular disease. It also restricts the emergence of chronic diseases such as cancer, Parkinson's and Alzheimer's.

Low calorie diets

Low-calorie diets include a reduction in the percentage of fat in the diet, thus reducing calories. Diet of this type includes NCEP Step I and II. A meta-analysis of 16 studies with a duration of 2 to 12 months indicates that low-calorie diets (without deliberately limiting calorie intake) result in an average weight loss of 3.2 kg (7.1 kg) compared to regular meals. Low calorie diets usually cause an energy deficit of 500-1,000 calories per day, which can result in 0.5kg (1.1kg) per 1kg (2.2kg) weight loss per week. Some of the most commonly used low-calorie diets are: Dash diet, Dieting diet and Weight Watchers.

Low Carbohydrate Diet

Low-carbohydrate diets (such as the Atkins diet) and protein diets have a relatively high protein content. A low-carbohydrate diet is sometimes called a keto diet (ie. they limit carbohydrate intake enough to cause ketosis). In the high-fat diet, only carbohydrates are restricted, with animal fat being the energy source. This was also the natural nutrition of man in antiquity.

Detoxifying diets

Detoxifying diets are thought to remove toxins from the body by increasing the amount of urine output, thus not giving the body enough time to digest the fat and toxins contained in everyday food.

Detoxifying diets often have side effects caused by the absence of these toxins during the first two or three days, which may include headache and drowsiness.

Detoxifying diets should never be started without first seeking medical advice.

Grandmothers always know!

Our grandmothers always knew what recipes and beauty tricks are natural and healthy, which has always been their advantage. They always have everything in the refrigerator, cabinet or basement, and they can mix up almost magical ointments and masks. That's why it's not surprising that their grandmothers have a favourite diet or rather a diet that has been word-of-mouth over the years.

Typically, for grandmothers, it does not include complete deprivation of some foods and starvation, but relies on pure foods and regular meals, but in smaller portions.

This diet has historical roots. The diet is practiced for over a decade by women in the world, as its results are really great: about four pounds can safely leave your body within a week. The main advantage of this diet is that it is a one-week course, and at your wish and need can be repeated two weeks later.

This diet is generally safe, but you must always keep in mind your health and emotional state before proceeding to any different diet regimen. It is advisable to consult with specialists as well.

Your daily schedule in keeping with the grandmother's diet should be as follows:

- Sleep is not less than 8 hours a day;

- The first breakfast should be no later than 30 minutes after awakening to warm the stomach and eliminate possible hunger spasms that will inevitably occur;

- Drink sour lemon juice or pure water during the day if you drink lemon juice, then immediately wash your mouth and teeth with bread soda. Lemon juice spoils the tooth enamel.

- Avoid all kinds of strong experiences, stress, scandals, quarrels, love thrills, and so on. Active physical exercises and exercises are also not desirable.

Seven days, use the following menu for this diet:

For breakfast: a cup of tea without sugar with lemon or fresh strawberries and freshly brewed black coffee;

Second breakfast: a piece of cheese weighing 40 grams;

Lunch: Meat, fried without butter in a pan or grilled - 120 g, boiled egg, cheese - 20 g, green salad;

After lunch: black coffee with milk or a glass of tea with lemon and fruit;

Dinner: Vegetable salad seasoned with vegetable oil and 120 grams boiled or stewed in own chicken meat sauce;

Mint is drunk at bedtime to eliminate stress in everyday life and a healthy sleep.

90 Day Diet - What is it?

One of the most popular diets on the web, especially among ladies.

The diet is partly based on the principle of segregated nutrition.

It is divided into four daily cycles, during which it is recommended to eat as follows:

Day 1: Protein - meat and dairy products, eggs, fish, vegetables

Day 2: Complex carbohydrates - legumes, cereals and root vegetables and vegetables

Day 3: Simple Carbohydrates - Sweets, cakes and more without the addition of milk and eggs are allowed, and for dinner - pastries, such as cakes, ice cream, chocolate

Day 4: Vitamins - only fruits, nuts and seeds, if you like, you can combine them with vegetables

Every 29 days there is a day of landing (for 90 days there are 3 in total). These days it is not allowed to eat, only pure non-carbonated water is consumed.

After the day of unloading you should follow a vitamin day and then a protein.

There are additional rules such as eating only between 12 and 20 hours, breakfast should consist of only fruits, the main meal is at lunch, and dinner should be 2 times less than lunch and more.

Why is the 90-day diet so popular and its application?

Diet, starting with a promise to loose between 15 and 25 pounds in 90 days, with no restrictions at all.

You can eat anything you want, including sweets, cakes, chocolate, pizza, etc., but only on certain days and hours.

Another reason it is so popular is that it is advertised by people rather than by a company trying to sell a product.

At the start, a drop in weight is quickly observed and enthusiastic about the quick result people share how much they have dropped and thus motivate others to do the same.

But the real effect I believe everybody is looking for is not just the lost weight, but the way we look.

Have you heard the words that the weight and what the scales are showing are not the most important how do we look in the mirror, and how do we feel in our own skin?

90 Day Diet - Shared Opinions

Everyone tells about what they have achieved, but how many people share the negative side of the coin on the other side of the coin?

Indeed, there are scientific studies that have calculated this ratio and it is 98: 2. (percentage share their results influenced by the positive emotion, against a percentage share their results after experiencing the negative from an event, combined with a shame of shame or worry about how they will look in the eyes of others).

When the popular diet is over, no one publicly tells how it feels, because often not only the body gets "cellulite" and / or stretch marks, but sometimes a lot of pounds or even all come back.

It turns out that a large number of people who have reached a late stage or who have completed the 90-day diet feel frustrated that no one shares the negatives of it but only the positive one.

However, I often get such messages, here is one of them: "I started the 90-day diet, I dropped 23 pounds. With me, the stretch marks are a lot, and before that I did not have any, something I think I could avoid with a healthy diet. I have stretch marks on my stomach, butt, chest, arms ... everything.

How does the 90-day diet work and does it work?

The answer is NO.

The reason for weight loss is the difference between calories consumed and those taken with food.

Typically, in a separate meal, dishes have a total reduced calorific value due to the exclusion of 1 macronutrient over a period of time.

Authors of books with separate diet recipes are mainly focused on dishes rich in vegetables, that is, with satiating effect and low caloric value.

Also, people who engage in such diets often have previously consumed unhealthy and high-calorie foods and beverages in inappropriate quantities.

The worse the eating habits a person had before the 90-day diet begins, the greater the kilogram amplitude will give.

Consideration should also be given to the fact that the observed loss of kilograms for the first few days is not burned fat.

The reason for the rapid loss of body weight is the limitations of carbohydrates and foods with added salt and sodium, which are the main responsible for the water balance and the storage of water in the body.

This is the reason why people think that eating from a separate meal is weakening.

Losing weight in this case is because of the calorie deficit and water handling, not because of the dietary intake.

Summary of the drawbacks of the 90-day diet

Lack of balance due to the many unjustified rules.

The diet supplies us with all types of nutrients, but on different days.

It is not a problem for our body to accept a variety of food at the same time and to process it, it is even advisable.

I will give an example of blood sugar. The richer the nutrients are given the nutrition, the lower the insulin response will be.

Loss of a small amount of muscle mass

People who decide to start the 90-day diet usually do not have a lot of muscle mass.

In a well-balanced diet, protein plays a major role, whereas in the 90-day diet, protein intake is once every four days.

This, combined with a negative caloric balance, guarantees significant muscle mass loss.

Yo-yo effect, stretch marks and cellulite.

Over 80% of people who lose weight with the 90-day diet then lose weight, but they have lost a lot of muscle mass, they've got loose skin, stretch marks and cellulite.

Something that makes the skin tight and tight, as well as giving shape to the body is exactly the muscle mass.

The basic idea of a good diet is to observe for a long time, to teach us about healthy habits and nutritional culture.

The shape and vision we are in is a reflection of our choices we make every day.

Returning to our old habits, we return to our old body.

Shortage of valuable vitamins and minerals.

Because each group of foods carries certain minerals it may be inadequate for the body to get them once every four days.

Not only because of the diluted intake, but also because of the quantities unrecognized by logic and research.

Vitamin C and B vitamins are water soluble. They are processed and disposed of permanently, so they need to be constantly stocked.

Options besides the 90-day diet

A smooth transition in calorie intake is a much healthier step than going from a non-compliance regime to a 90-day diet.

The first step you can take is to enter small, healthy replacements.

Such replacements are:

• Drinking more water instead of other beverages (over 3 liters);

- Stew sweetener and cinnamon instead of sugar;

- Whole fruit instead of natural or squeezed juice;

- Oat pancakes instead of flour;

- A glass of red wine instead of beer or a calorie cocktail;

- Whole grains instead of redesigned versions;

- Oatmeal instead of muesli and cereal mixes;

- Mustard instead of mayonnaise;

- Raw nuts instead of roasted with added salt;

- Charlotte (more accessible version) or olive oil instead of refined oil;

- More often roast and boiled instead of fried;

- Mix spices and potassium / Himalayan salt instead of plain;

- Rice instead of chips or snacks;

- Consumption of food as much as you feel, not until the dish is empty.

These small replacements would be more than enough to move things in a positive direction, but without the stress, limitations and possible unwanted side effects of the 90-day diet.

You will also lose weight at the beginning - again, as mentioned earlier in the article, because of the reduction in salt and sodium, which are the main responsible for the balance and the amount of stored water in the body.

But at the same time you will feel more vibrant and energetic, weight loss will be healthier, you will not lose a big percentage of your muscle mass and then, if you wish, you will easily build on what you have achieved.

Because after you have finished the ninety-day diet that puts you in such constraints, and it turns out you have not achieved the desired results, what's next? Another 90-day diet?

17 foods that kill the appetite

Appetite is the desire to consume food, but this desire is not always related to hunger. He is responsible for adequate energy intake in order to maintain the metabolic needs of the body. Appetite can also be stimulated by food of good taste, smell, appearance and others without being hungry. Also under stress his levels increase and this easily leads to uncontrolled food intake.

The good news is that there are foods that have proven appetite suppression properties and can help make it easier to maintain good shape.

1. Spicy red pepper

Hot pepper contains an ingredient called capsaicin.

There are studies that have established the link between capsaicin and appetite suppression.

Capsaicin has thermo-genetic properties, which means it can raise the temperature and lead to an increase in blood flow and acceleration of the metabolism.

Cold red pepper is also used in food burn supplements, which is another proof of its effectiveness.

2. Cinnamon

In a cinnamon-based study, participants are asked to add 6 grams of cinnamon in a rice pudding to see if it has an effect on appetite suppression.

It was concluded that cinnamon slows the absorption of carbohydrates from the small intestine. Participants who used cinnamon felt better than those who consumed cinnamon-free pudding.

Cinnamon has the fame of spice, which works to lower subcutaneous fat and lose weight. Although there is no direct effect on accelerating metabolism or on burning calories, the main benefit comes from the property and regulates blood sugar.

Cinnamon can be added to rice, yoghurt, hot drinks, soups, fruits, meats, and more.

Other spices that are known for their blood glucose control properties are cloves and ginger.

3. Nuts

Nuts contain beneficial fats, protein, carbohydrate with low glycemic index and fibre, which releases energy slowly into the body and keep it sated for a long time.

It should be kept in mind that nuts are calorie foods. 30 grams of raw almonds contain 160 calories, 14 grams of fat, 6 grams of carbohydrate (3 fibres), 6 grams of protein.

4. Avocado

Avocado contains healthy monounsaturated fats, which are absorbed slowly and satiated for a long time. It is also an excellent source of soluble fibre, which forms a thick gel in the presence of a liquid. This process slows absorption and clears the intestine, and thus affects cholesterol lowering.

Avocados is also a calorie diet. A medium avocado (200 grams) contains: 320 calories, 30 grams of fat, 17 grams of carbohydrates (13 fibres) and 4 grams of protein. Of the 30 grams of fat, about 20 are monounsaturated.

5. Black chocolate

Good news for all chocolate lovers!

According to recent studies, black chocolate has a number of beneficial properties, and with regular consumption it is almost certain that you will lose weight.

Not only will it help to lose weight in your abdomen and reduce your waist by at least 4 sm, but it's too good to be true. Do not believe everything you read on the web, think about the information you get, and the different points of view.

The information, which states that black chocolate is "useful", is based on studies of the type (the two studies are quite real):

Study I: A study of white and black chocolate and their effects on blood sugar found that participants who consumed black chocolate had lower blood sugar than those who consumed white chocolate.

Study II: A study found that participants who consumed black chocolate some time before a main meal (exemplified by pizza) ate 15% less pizza than those who ate milk chocolate.

It can be concluded that black chocolate is "less evil" than white or milky, but at the same time a 70% (100 g) Lindt chocolate contains: 625 calories, 47 g Fat, 30 g saturated fat , 25 mg. Sodium, 7.5 g Fibre, 42 g Carbohydrates, 30 g of Sugar and 7.5 g of Protein.

6. Flaxseed

Flax seed is rich in fibre and omega 3 fatty acids, and is also a source of protein. A Danish study found that supplementing with 2.5 grams of linseed per day had a positive effect on appetite suppression compared to another group given a placebo supplement.

Our bodies cannot absorb the flax seed. It needs to be broken beforehand in order to get all the benefits from it. It can be stored in a freezer for better storage of omega 3 fatty acids. You can add a spoon of flaxseed to oatmeal, yoghurt, salad or protein shake.

7. Oat nuts

Oatmeal is a well-balanced diet suitable for both weight loss and weight gain.

They have a high fibre content, which means they will keep you sit for a longer time.

Complex carbohydrates have a low glycemic index, which means you will get a slow and gradual release of energy without having a particular effect on blood sugar and therefore fat deposition.

If you're one of the people who are constantly feeling hungry, plugging oatmeal into your daily menu would definitely help if breakfast is not the only place they can attend.

8. Apples

Apples contain a kind of soluble fibre called pectin.

Pectin reduces the amount of sugar absorbed by the bloodstream after a meal, preventing large increases in blood sugar, which would lead to fat storage as well as the need for sweet foods.

Apple combines perfectly with cinnamon and can hold you sit for up to 2 hours.

9. Beans

Beans, lentils, peas, chickpeas and others are a good source of vegetarian protein. Rich in soluble fibre as well as complex carbohydrates, called oligosaccharides. Like fibre, these carbohydrates are not absorbed by the body, and this slows down digestion, thus keeping us longer for a long time.

Studies have shown that beans can help reduce appetite and chemical levels - compounds called typein inhibitors and lectins, promoting the release of a hormone called cholecystokinin, which slows the emptying of our stomach and keeps us longer for a long time.

10.Cottage cheese

Not surprisingly, skimmed cottage cheese is a healthy choice for people on diet and fitness enthusiasts. It is low in fat and carbohydrates (almost zero) and is a rich source of complete protein. Casein in skimmed cottage cheese can suppress appetite.

The curd can be combined well with omelettes or black / red pepper and onion.

11.Meat

The high protein content of the meat and the presence of saturated fat is a prerequisite for a slower digestion of the food. Meat takes more time to chew, which also helps to create a feeling of satiety.

Numerous studies have shown that there is no difference between chicken, veal, pork and other meats in terms of what saturation they contribute if they are similar in composition to proteins and fats.

12.Green vegetables

Vegetable vegetables are of utmost importance for any well-balanced diet. They contain good amounts of vitamins, minerals, antioxidants and other nutrients.

The topic - high water and fibre content will help to achieve satiety for longer. Also, vegetables require time to consume - the act of slow chewing also helps. It takes about 15-20 minutes to synthesize a hormone that sends signals to the brain for satiety.

Part of the leafy greens are spinach, parsley, dock, broccoli and others.

13.Green tea

Like coffee, green tea also has the ability to speed up metabolism. Contains natural antioxidants, called polyphenols, that have a beneficial effect on glucose levels and insulin sensitivity.

Consumption of green tea increases the release of the cholecystokinin hormone (which was mentioned in legumes), sending a signal to the brain for satiety.

Green tea has a pleasant taste. Another way it can be useful is as an alternative to calorie drinks and limiting excess meals.

14.Coffee

In moderate amounts, coffee can have a good effect on health. An excellent ingredient when our goal is to burn excess fat and speed up our metabolism.

At the same time, there are good appetite suppressants. Drinking a cup of coffee can reduce the desire to eat in the short term.

Caffeine has a number of health benefits, but its excessive consumption can affect hormonal imbalance, headache, anxiety and insomnia.

If you decide to use coffee as a suppressant, be sure to drink pure coffee. For example Starbucks coffee can reach up to 400 calories, mainly from fat and sugars, and only one cup.

15.Water

Although water passes quickly through the digestive system, it can help reduce appetite in several ways. It has been proven that hunger and thirst signals are very close, and the reason we experience hunger is, in fact, often due to dehydration.

Cold water consumption is also warmed up to body temperature in the body and thus speeds up metabolism for a short time, which in turn burns extra calories. If you weigh 70 kilograms, the healthy amount of water would be between 2.5 - 4 litres of water per day. When determining what limit to choose, consider: climate, physical activity and sweating.

16. Apple vinegar

Natural apple vinegar has proven properties in regulating blood sugar and, therefore, at weight loss and overall health.

In one study, the participants took a natural apple vinegar with carbohydrates in the form of white bread.

Blood tests have shown that the group that received apple vinegar has lower blood sugar and insulin levels than other participants.

17. Coconut oil

Coconut oil is one of the best choices for high temperature cooking. It can also be added to coffee, tea, salad dressing, troubles, and more.

Coconut oil contains mostly medium chain triglycerides (MCFA), unlike other cooking oils, which contain mainly long chain triglycerides.

Some studies have shown that medium-chain triglycerides have the properties of oxidizing in the liver, which means that some of them will most likely be used as fuel.

However, it should be kept in mind that coconut oil is calorie and should be used in moderate amounts.

Plus Quality Sleep

The link between lack of quality sleep and low levels of the hormone leptin - a hormone that controls appetite, has been proven, while the levels of the hormone responsible for the stimulation of hunger - ghirlin are rising.

Not surprisingly, people with poor sleep usually have problems with their eating habits.

Healthy Eating: The Best Diet

What defines healthy eating?

Every answer to this question is different, but in the broadest sense of healthy eating is considered the consumption of foods from different groups that make us feel good, have more energy, better mood and maintain or improve your health.

Healthy eating is certainly not a rigorous diet and limitation that promises quick results for a short time (an example is the 90-day diet) or makes you deprive 100% of the foods you love.

Diet is often associated with overweight removal but is actually the food we consume within 24 hours, one week, one month or another time.

It is a good diet that promotes good and optimal health.

It should include several groups of foods because a single group can not provide everything (protein, carbohydrate, fat, fibre, vitamin and minerals) from which a human organism needs.

A healthy diet combined with physical activity is considered to be the safest and most reliable way to reduce the risk of disease in the long term and to reach or maintain optimal weight and beautiful vision.

If you feel overwhelmed by the whole conflict of opinions on the internet, when it comes to healthy eating and dieting, you are not alone.

It seems that behind every opinion that a diet or diet is good and appropriate, there is at least one other opinion, which claims the opposite.

With this healthy eating guide, you can remove confusing tips to create a delicious, varied and healthy diet that is good for both your body and your mind.

How to eat healthy?

For most people who do not have food allergies, this can happen by focusing on the following foods:

• Pure meat (without skin / cut-off fat) - mainly sources of protein;

• Fish (such as salmon, trout, herring) - mainly sources of protein, unsaturated and omega 3 fat;

• Variety of vegetables - sources of fibre, vitamins and minerals;

• Whole grains (such as oatmeal, brown rice and wild rice) - sources mainly of complex carbohydrates, vitamins and minerals;

• Raw nuts and seeds (almonds, hazelnuts, peanuts and flax, sunflower, buckwheat) - mainly sources of fat, vitamins and minerals;

• Vegetable protein (like beans and lentils) - mainly sources of complex carbohydrates, fibre and protein;

• Limited quantities of fruit (why is a restriction in fruit?) - sources of mainly fibre, vitamins and minerals;

• Limited quantities of dairy products. - sources of vitamins, minerals and a balanced amount of protein, carbohydrate and fat.

As you may notice, when a meal is not altered artificially, it does not only contain proteins, only carbohydrates or only fat.

It is believed that this is one of the reasons that these foods act so well on our body and allow for positive health changes, no matter what our goals are.

One of the many benefits of unprocessed foods is that supplying different types of nutrients and micronutrients (vitamins and minerals) slows down the rise in blood sugar (usually when consuming highly processed foods).

A regular rise in blood sugar, in turn, is associated with fat storage and excess weight gain, a rapid drop in energy and tonus after eating, a risk of illness such as diabetes, and so on.

What to drink?

Water consumption also plays a key role when talking about healthy eating. In fact, excessive consumption of drinks with added sugar and other enhancers have failed a diet or diet.

If you need to add flavour to your water, add a slice of lemon, lime, cucumber or natural tea.

Coffee can also be a good option if you are not too sensitive to it and do not interfere with your day-to-day activities or sleep.

Even in dietary supplements for weight loss, caffeine is often an essential ingredient and may be useful if our goal is extra fat burning

When we eat, it also matters (sometimes).

Everywhere you can read tips such as breakfast is the most important meal, and that the last meal should be light and not contain a particular type of food.

Recent studies, however, prove the claim that it does not matter whether we consume the largest portion of food in the morning, at noon or in the evening.

An institution who conducted one of these studies in charge of weight control: "It does not matter at what time of day you eat. It is important to know what amounts are taken and the physical activity you make throughout the day. They will determine whether you will increase, lose or save your weight. "

Of course, even and more frequent meals have their health benefits (not morning or evening).

How much food we will consume and how it will be distributed depends mostly on physical activity, and when there is no physical activity, even distribution is the most appropriate option.

Regular consumption of food is the best way to optimize your body's energy levels, provided that the total number of calories per day meets the set goals (maintenance, weight gain or weight reduction).

This is because it creates an environment where there are no extreme increases and decreases in blood sugar levels, which in turn has a direct connection with the energy available to the body.

Accordingly, in severe physical activities, it is logical to emphasize more nutrients in the range before and after.

The health benefits associated with more frequent nutrition are: optimal energy levels, effective blood sugar regulation, better nutrition, especially protein, better control of the feeling of sweet or uncontrollable appetite.

Feeding before sleep

Until a few years ago, it was believed that after 6 or 8 pm. it was bad to consume food or that before sleep that consumption would immediately affect our weight.

Serious researches, as well as fitness enthusiasts in personal blogs and YouTube, have done a number of experiments consuming most of their carbohydrates for the day just before bedtime and have once again achieved a loss of excess fat.

The conclusion is that this is not, in fact, the most important and necessary factor on which to make great effort and energy when we can concentrate on much more important things.

In fact, eating before sleep has some benefits:

1. Regulate blood sugar throughout the day, but mostly in the morning;

2. Regular consumption of quality and healthy food at bedtime will help to avoid unexpected meals at night and early in the morning;

3. Can improve the quality of sleep because you will not try to fall asleep, nor will you wake up hungry at night.

Consuming quality food at bedtime is actually much healthier than waking up at night to consume junk food or unhealthy breakfast after getting up.

It is recommended that the last meal be at 6 pm. because it was believed that by 8 to 9 pm. you would already be in bed.

One of the most damaging things you can do about your metabolism, your optimal weight and your health as a whole: Last meal at 6pm, fall asleep at 11-12 am. , wake up at 8-9, skip breakfast and you make your first meal at 1-2 pm., which is usually an unhealthy option.

In this way, they collect about 15 hours without food.

But we all know that, in fact, between these hours, unhealthy foods are most often consumed, and you wonder why you have such a need, and you cannot give up.

Read this paragraph again and you will answer the question, and whether you will take action depends only on you.

However, there is a group of foods that should be avoided at bedtime and these are the processed foods and fruits because of the amount of sugar they contain.

It is believed that sugar prevents the release of the growth hormone, which naturally synthesizes in the greatest quantities during a deep sleep.

Basics of Healthy Eating - What to Have at Your Hand

You may have heard the phrase "If you fail in planning, you are planning your failure."

This is one of my favourite tips when it comes to healthy eating, diets and fitness as a whole.

With the hectic daily routine and long working days, it is much easier to make quick and easy choices, even to realize that they are not the best for us.

Therefore, stocking healthy foods is the key to sticking to pre-set prices - be it healthy eating, weight loss or more.

Prepared with the right foods, it will be much easier for you after a long and exhausting day, instead of making a phone call and ordering fast food, doing something delicious and healthy at home.

So not just that the food will contain what you need, and in most cases you will save time and money.

Foods to keep in the cabinets

These are foods that do not spoil and can be used in a variety of combinations to prepare a quick and healthy meal.

- Oat flakes;

- Whole grains (rice, spaghetti, macaroni, etc.);

- Canned beans - some variants have added sugar, but most contain beans, water and salt;

- Canned tuna in own sauce;

- Spices - cinnamon, ginger, red and pepper, cumin, etc .;

• Raw nuts - almonds, walnuts, peanuts, hazelnuts, Brazil nuts, etc .;

• Seeds - Flaxseed, Chia Seeds, Pumpkin Seeds, Sesame Seeds, Sunflower Seeds, etc.

Foods to charge the refrigerator

When you get hungry, the first place you check for food is usually the refrigerator.

Opening the fridge make sure you have at least a few of the listed foods:

• Eggs - all the vitamins and minerals we need, quality protein and useful fat;

• Degreased curd - a source of quality protein with 0% fat and 0% carbohydrates, minimum calories;

• Yogurt - balanced food containing all macronutrients;

• Skimmed or low-fat milk - a source of calcium, potassium and vitamin D, essential nutrients for our bodies;

• Mustard - a good substitute for popular high-calorie options. Make sure you buy an option without added sugar.

Foods to charge the fridge

• Vegetables and fruits - a perfect addition to any meal, soup, turmoil or other shake;

• Shrimps - because they are small in volume, thawing and cooking do not take long;

• Meat and fish - chicken breast, turkey bon fillet, trout and others.

Adding at least part of the listed foods combined with the removal of some of the unhealthy choices (such as over-processed foods) is taking a big step on the way to healthy eating.

What cooking oils do we use?

• Coconut oil - the winner of the fat-containing rating that can be used to power our bodies similarly to carbohydrates.

• Avocado oil - avocado oil, just like coconut, is suitable for cooking and does not lose its nutritional value and its beneficial substances on heating.

• Olive oil - high nutritional value, cold pressed and unrefined products, but lose most of the useful substances in heating. A significantly cheaper alternative to coconut oil and avocado oil.

How to make a healthy meal part of our lives?

Set up correctly to succeed

Changing much of your habits that you have built up for years is almost a sure path to failure.

To make sure you stick to healthier habits, try to think long-term.

This can happen by taking small steps that do not burden you physically and mentally and which you think will be able to perform over a prolonged period of time.

When a few small steps become a habit, then you can add even more healthy choices.

To this column we can also add:

• Prepare much of your food at home - This will allow better control of food quality and calorie intake;

• If you do not want to count strictly calories, concentrate on healthy substitutions (many of which are described at the end of the article for the 90-day diet), as well as on variety, freshness and color in the choice of foods. This in itself involves the avoidance of packaged and processed foods;

• Read labels - It is extremely important to know what you are buying. Many manufacturers manage to hide harmful ingredients under different names, even in products that are advertised as healthy.

• Pay attention to how you feel after eating - Often while eating junk food, we do not think that after a few minutes we may experience unwanted effects - physically and mentally like stomach discomfort, sorry for the large number of calories consumed, etc.

• Consume more water - Helps purify from waste products and toxins that cause fatigue, lack of energy, headaches, etc. It has been found that in most cases the feeling of thirst can be confused with that of hunger, so good hydration will help make healthier choices.

Give your body more often what you need

In most cases, after most of your meals you have to feel satisfied, but do not overwhelm.

Do not exclude completely favourite food groups. Thus, while healthy, change is often short-lived, and if you are tempted, you will feel as if you have failed.

An option you can try is to reduce the amount of unhealthy food (for example, in half) and to consume less often during the week.

When trying to lose excess weight, slowing, as well as stopping shortly before you are fully fed, can have very big benefits in controlling calories. The reason is that it takes a few minutes to pass the required signals for satiety at a chemical level.

Limit your sugar and salt consumption, but do not replace it with unhealthy choices

Sugar

Excessive consumption of sugar causes inconsistent levels of energy and is associated with diabetes, depression and an increase in unhealthy weight.

Reducing sugar from desserts is only part of the solution, as the amount of added sugar is in bread, muesli, canned fruits and vegetables, sauces, margarine, potato puree (something that is used in most restaurants instead of real potatoes), frozen foods, foods with reduced natural fat, fast food, ketchup and more.

Our bodies can get the sugar they need from natural sources such as fruits, so that everything listed is often too many calories that have no nutritional value and beneficial effect.

Some tips to help reduce sugar:

• Reduce the sugar in the daily menu gradually;

• Avoid spirits;

• Do not replace saturated fat with sugar (eg low-fat milk with "fruit / berries");

• Avoid processed and packaged foods;

• When dining out, keep in mind that most sauces and dressings are supplemented with large amounts of sugar and salt because restaurants are only interested in providing a better flavour.

Salt

Salt is another ingredient that is often used over recommended daily values to improve the taste of a dish or drink.

Our bodies need about 8-15 grams of salt per day to function optimally (or 1/2 to 1 tablespoon).

Consumption of large amounts of salt is associated with high blood pressure and water retention. Greater misuse may lead to an increased risk of stroke, heart and kidney disease, memory loss and erectile dysfunction.

Here are some tips to help reduce salt:

• Processed and packaged foods often contain a high amount of sodium and one meal may exceed the daily recommended intake;

• Use more natural spices such as garlic, curry, black pepper and red pepper to improve the taste of dishes;

• When eating out, keep in mind that most foods contain high amounts of salt. You may want to pre-add and flavour your food yourself.

Consequences of unhealthy eating

A lot of people are overweight or obese according to the body mass index, but only 35% think they are thicker than normal. Despite the serious health consequences, people still cannot realize the importance of these problems.

This shows the results of a National Survey of Overweight of the MBMD Sociological Agency, commissioned by the pharmaceutical company Roche.

According to studies at least 200,000 people die prematurely each year as a result of stroke, heart disease and other illnesses associated with an unhealthy diet.

Also, many of those who do not die prematurely do not enjoy painless old age, no limitation and disability.

It is claimed that over 80% of the population consumes excessive amounts of salt. Something that most do not realize is that over 75% of the body's required salt is added in advance to food, even without salting their meals.

Nutritionists claim that 3/4 of all cancers can be prevented through healthy eating and proper diet. A healthy diet can protect you from diabetes, osteoporosis, cardiovascular disease, stroke, etc., and help you feel better every day.

Conclusion

As you may have noticed, no severe calorie restriction or starvation is recommended to reduce or maintain optimal weight and good health.

Instead, I believe that if you have no dietary experience, it is most rational to gradually add healthy foods, excluding unhealthy (again gradually) from your diet.

By combining the tips in the article with exercises several times a week, the desired results will not be delayed.

Cellulite: How to deal with the eternal problem – Cellulite

Cellulite (also called lipodystrophy) is an uneven build up of subcutaneous fat, which gives the skin a faint look. It occurs most often in the pelvic region (especially the buttocks), legs and abdomen. Cellulite has most women who have had in puberty. Research shows that it is present in 85-90% of women, which means that it is a physiological phenomenon rather than pathological. It can be due to a complex combination of factors - from hormones to heredity.

Reasons

Causes of cellulite include changes in metabolism, physiology, diet and habits, as well as obesity, changes in connective tissue structure, hormonal factors and genetic factors.

Kinds

The various classifications of skin deformities called cellulitis are related to the change in structure, consistency and localization. In general, according to the sensation of gripping the skin, the cellulite is divided into "soft" and "hard", but often there is added a third - "swollen". Besides these species, they can also meet sclerosing, adipose, local, compact, sporty.

Cellulite treatment

Cellulite is a multifactorial condition that is resistant to a wide range of methods of treatment. However, there are treatment options, such as regular skin care, following a strict diet to reduce excess fat, and massages.

What are the reasons for the appearance of cellulite?

Cellulite has been common in all people and has been observed since ancient times, but the reasons for its occurrence are controversial. These include diet, accumulation of toxins in the body, genetic heritage, skin thickness, the amount and distribution of body fat, hormonal balance, and age.

Here are some details of the most common reasons.

Way of eating

People who consume too much fat, carbohydrates and salt and too little fibre are more likely to develop cellulite. Dairy products and carbonated beverages make it worse when it's already there.

Lifestyle

Cellulite is more common in smokers and people with a stale lifestyle.

Much less cellulite has people who exercise regularly.

A fitness program that focuses on areas with cellulite - buttocks, thighs, abdomen has a positive influence.

Underwear

Wearing low-elastic underwear in the back may reduce blood flow and increase the risk of cellulite formation.

Extra pounds and pregnancy

Cellulite is more common in overweight people. Subcutaneous fat levels increase and this leads to greater pressure on the connective tissue.

Reducing excess weight always has a positive effect on cellulite.

Age and hereditary factors

The risk of developing cellulite increases with age. The likelihood of cellulite appears to increase gradually after the age of 25 and may occur relatively early in people with genetic predisposition.

How to Get Rid of Cellulite?

Cellulite is a cosmetic problem. Although it may be a symptom of other health problems such as obesity and predisposition to genetically transmitted diseases, its treatment should not always be ambulatory.

Here are some proven ways to deal with cellulite, ranging from the shortest to the longest.

Creams for spreading

They are the most popular way to deal with cellulite because they are easy to use. However, it is important to know that their efficacy is limited. The reason for this is in their local application.

Here's the long explanation:

The most common active ingredients in anti-cellulite creams are called methylxanthines.

These are a group of chemicals that include aminophylline, caffeine and theophylline.

These chemicals can be found in most creams because of their known ability to break down fatty deposits.

However, creams for topical application on cellulite skin cannot provide the necessary concentration of these chemicals for the time required for significant decomposition of subcutaneous fat.

Studies have shown that creams containing methylxanthines have an effect, but their benefit is not recommended for sustained release from cellulite.

Another popular active ingredient in anti-cellulite shaves is retinol or vitamin A1. Retinol is used in facial skin wrinkles. When used no less than twice a day, it can be expected to smooth out the cellulite skin after about 6 months.

Massage therapy

There are two types of anti-cellulite massage: manual and machine. In both cases, the massage is local and is performed on areas affected by cellulite.

Rolling cylinders are used in machine massage, which pulls and presses against each other of the skin and massages them in a special mini-camera. A good example of such massage therapy is Endermologie, developed in France and used to treat cellulite since the mid-1990s.

This technique uses a power supply device that sucks, pulls and presses affected areas. The procedure lasts 30-45 minutes and typically requires between 10 and 12 sessions before the results become noticeable. The temporary reduction in cellulite has been proven, but the technique is expensive and often reallocates fat instead of permanently changing the fat-tissue configuration under the skin.

Regular treatment is needed to maintain the initial effect or cellulite will inevitably return.

Some doctors connect cellulite to the lymphatic system. They recommend two types of massage treatment for cellulite: deep-tissue massage and scrub massage. These procedures stimulate lymphatic glands and improve blood flow.

To improve the efficiency of the scrub, you can dip it into a mixture of algae and olive oil. This will improve its lymphatic effect, but with all the decisions so far, and it is short-lived and should be done periodically to produce results.

Laser therapy

This is a low-invasive ambulatory technique approved in the United States by the US Food and Drug Administration in 2015. Under subcision, a dermatologist places a needle under the skin that breaks down the connective tissue fibres. The results last about 2 years, after which reintroduction may be necessary. The most effective sites for cellulite subcision are in the thighs.

There are other sanitary methods, such as laser surgery combined with suction, as well as laser therapy combined with machine massages, but these procedures are really very expensive.

Weight loss through diet and workouts

Although cellulite can occur in weak people, it is much less common than in overweight people.

As we have already explained, cellulite appears when the adipose tissue presses the connective fibres of the skin.

Movement and exercise are the most effective way to burn excess fat. Fewer fats lead to less fat tissue that presses the connective tissue.

Indeed, there is no longer-term solution to prevent and eliminate cellulite from weight loss through training and proper nutrition.

Focus on foods rich in fibre and limit fat and carbohydrates. Start attending a fitness club twice a week and combine with classical and tried-and-tested methods to fight cellulite such as creams for spreading.

It may take a while, but you will not find a more durable method for dealing with cellulite.

The result will not just deliver you from cellulite, but it will also make you fall in love again in your body.

Are you struggling with cellulite and by what methods? What has helped you so far?

Protein: The Most Tasty and Healthy Way to Weight Loss

Proteins (proteins) are basic building blocks in the cellular structures of living organisms. The main thing to remember is their role in our nutrition - to help the human body to renew, grow and develop.

The full functioning of the human body requires the consumption of a certain amount of amino acids every day. They get it by digesting the proteins (protein) in the food and digesting the amino acids that make up the proteins.

If the amount of protein in human food is permanently low, the body reacts with slow growth, loss of muscle and body mass (eats), illness and even death.

After this short presentation, the main question is:

How can protein intake help to lose weight?

Protein is the most important nutrient for losing weight and achieving a good-looking body.

High protein intake has been shown to accelerate metabolism, reduce appetite, and positively affect hormones that are closely related to weight regulation, such as ghrelin, GIP and GLP-1 (satiety hormones).

The protein will help in weight loss and fat loss even in the most problematic areas through many actions and mechanisms.

In this article you will learn about the effects of protein on weight loss and weight loss.

The protein changes the levels of several hormone-regulating hormones

Weight is actively regulated by the brain, especially in the area called hypothalamus.

In order for the brain to determine exactly when and how much to eat, it processes many different information.

Some of the most important signals to the brain are hormones that change in response to nutrition.

Higher protein intake has been shown to increase levels of GLP-1 and cholecystokinin (hormones that suppress appetite and are of great importance for weight loss) while reducing the ghrelin hormone (at high levels, we feel hunger and low levels suppress and regulates appetite).

When we take larger amounts of protein, we will naturally lower the amounts of carbohydrates and fats.

These are two different mechanisms with which the protein will help in weight loss and weight loss.

Professional advice: When aiming at weight loss, I recommend consuming protein sources at the beginning of your meals with vegetables and water. This will reduce the intake of other more calorie choices.

Briefly: The protein effectively regulates the levels of hormones that are responsible for appetite and hunger. At the same time, higher protein intake naturally reduces other macronutrients (fat, carbohydrates), thus automatically taking fewer calories - 2 different mechanisms that will help you lose weight.

Digestion and protein metabolism burn calories

Following food intake, processes in the body start as digestion and metabolism.

These processes are known as "thermal effects of food".

Although different sources differ in terms of exact figures, it has been shown that protein has the highest thermal effect (between 20-30%) compared to carbohydrates (5-10%) and fats (0-3%).

Assuming the thermal effect of the protein is 30%, it means that of the 100 calories provided by the protein source only 70 will be usable.

Professional advice: When preparing a nutritional plan, take a higher percentage of calories from proteins as they have the highest thermal effect.

Briefly: About 20-30% of the calories taken from protein sources are burned while the body grinds and metabolizes the protein.

The protein helps you burn more calories at rest (until you are not physically active)

This effect causes the body to burn more calories throughout the day, even during sleep.

Several studies have shown that high protein intake speeds up metabolism and increases the amount of calories burned by 80-100 every day (1) (2) (3).

This effect is even more pronounced if you follow a diet to increase muscle mass or you are in a big calorie surplus. Burned calories from increased protein intake may reach ~ 260 per day.

Professional advice: As the last meal of the day, choose a source of protein and useful fat. This will slow the flow of amino acids to the blood and thus provide your body with valuable nutrients throughout the night.

Do not take sugar, even if it is fruity or honey. This will prevent the release of growth hormone - a hormone associated with increased fat burning, rejuvenation, weight reduction and other benefits.

Briefly: Higher protein intake can burn between 80 and 100 calories a day, burning is not associated with physical activity, but with the amount of protein intake (more = more calories burned).

Protein reduces appetite and makes you consume fewer calories

Protein can reduce hunger and appetite by several different mechanisms.

This in turn will automatically reduce your daily caloric intake.

In other words, even if you do not keep track of how many calories you take (something I strongly recommend) or do not control your portions consciously, you will eventually consume less food and calories.

A number of studies have shown that when people increase protein intake, they start to consume fewer calories, both in individual meals and throughout the day.

This effect is sometimes more pronounced if they have not previously adhered to healthy eating habits and specialized guidelines.

In this study (English), increasing protein consumption by 30% has reduced the intake of an average of 441 calories a day, which is a huge amount.

Example: 30 minutes of cardio workout on a trail, fast walking on a slope will burn about 300 calories.

High protein diets, not only have a metabolic advantage, but also a great advantage in controlling and regulating appetite, against diets that restrict protein intake.

Professional advice: High protein diet often restricts other macronutrients, such as carbohydrates.

To compensate for this restriction and to regulate appetite, add a large portion of vegetables (cucumbers, peppers, broccoli, zucchini, cauliflower, spinach, mushrooms, lettuce, onions, garlic, etc.) with natural green tea.

In short: High protein diets have a strong satiating effect and lead to reduction and easy control of appetite, especially when compared to low protein regimens. This makes it much easier to consume fewer calories in each meal and thus easier weight loss and weight reduction.

Protein reduces the desire for unhealthy intermediate meals

The uncontrollable desire for unhealthy meals between main meals and at night is one of the main causes of diet failure.

Many people gain weight because of the tendency to consume too much food late at night or when they wake up occasionally.

The most common reason for this is the lack of nutrients and macronutrients (mostly carbohydrates), as well as poor distribution of food and calories throughout the day.

For joy, increased protein intake is directly linked to a decrease in the desire for unhealthy eating and the consumption of too many calories at night / at night.

This study (English) compares a high protein diet with a moderate protein diet in overweight men.

The high protein group reduced the desire for additional meals by 60% and the desire to eat at night, half.

Professional advice: Breakfast is one of the most important meals to load your body with protein. The reasons are several:

• This will allow you to make a healthy first meal by taking the most of your calories from good sources;

• This way you can turn off carbohydrates from the first meal or at least reduce them as a quantity. This will keep your blood sugar levels at a moderate level. This is one of the strongest prerequisites and the most beneficial environment for burning fat;

• You will start the day loaded with tone and energy, and with the satisfaction that you have done something for yourself. Often at a bad start of the day, we tend to go on as we started, is it familiar to you?

In Brief: Consumption of more protein leads to a significant reduction in the desire for unhealthy small meals and for starvation late at night. This in turn will make it much easier to stick to a diet or diet.

Increased intake of protein helps to lose weight, even if you do not consciously restrict your caloric intake

The protein works on both sides of the "Calories Accepted Against Burned Calories". Its intake reduces the accepted calories while boosting the burned.

For this reason, it is no surprise that high protein diets can lead to weight loss, even without limiting conscious calories, portions, fats, or carbohydrates.

In a study conducted with 19 overweight people, increasing the protein intake by 30% resulted in a significant decrease in caloric intake (link to the study).

This study shows how average participants lost 11 pounds over a 12-week period. They are said to have added protein to their diet, but they have not intentionally constrained anything else.

Although the results are not always so dramatic, most of the studies show that high protein diets lead to significant weight loss.

Higher protein intake is also associated with less fat around the abdomen and less "harmful fats" that accumulate around the human organs and can cause illnesses.

Despite all of the above, weight loss is not the only and most important factor. It is even more important to keep the results.

Many people manage to start a diet and lose weight, but most of them return much of what they have achieved (more than 90% of Google's query), and there are even cases where the end result is more pounds than the start point.

Higher protein intake may help prevent the recovery of an unhealthy weight.

So moderate or high intake of protein may not only help you when you are aiming at weight loss but also prevent loss of results already achieved, especially when combined with exercise.

Professional advice: After completing a diet or diet, even return to your previous habits try to maintain high intake of protein. This will greatly help to preserve the results achieved.

In short: Taking more protein can lead to weight loss even without counting the calories you eat (something that I strongly recommend (2)), portions control, or additional restrictions on carbohydrate and fat intake. A minimal increase in protein intake is also associated with a greater chance of retaining results already achieved after a diet or diet.

Protein helps to prevent muscle loss and metabolism delays

Losing weight is never equal to fat loss alone.

At weight loss, the muscle mass also decreases.

But what you really want to lose is subcutaneous fat (under the skin) and visceral fat (fat around the organs).

Losing muscle mass is a side effect that accompanies weight loss. Most people do not realize the unpleasant visual effects that follow after losing the little muscle they have and therefore do not make any effort in that direction.

Another common effect of weight loss, which comes mostly from an aggressive restriction in caloric intake, is the slowing down of the metabolism (metabolism in the body).

In other words, the body will start burning fewer calories and will make it harder to lose weight.

I started writing ... "It will make it harder to lose weight, regardless of whether you reduce your calories," but in fact it is possible that even the moment when the more and more aggressively you reduce your calories, the less the body burns .

In the gym, this effect is known as switching to sleep mode and can prevent hundreds of calories burning each day.

In this way, weight loss becomes practically impossible if you do not completely change your approach. This is one of the reasons why we often hear phrases such as "I eat nothing, but I do not lose weight"

Taking larger amounts of protein will reduce muscle loss, which will limit your metabolic damage even with more restrictive diets.

Exercises and weight training (even minimal ones) are also a major factor in maintaining muscle mass and effectively working metabolism.

For this reason, the high protein content in your diet and strength training are two crucial components for achieving long-term results for a primary goal of weight loss.

The combination of high protein intake and strength training has another huge plus. Without them, there is a great chance of getting disappointed with the final result, even if you achieve the desired weight loss in kilograms.

The reason is that what tightens the body and gives it a beautiful shape is actually a mass of mass (a combination of muscle mass and fat in a given ratio). After you lose weight and burn fat, if you do not have the already mentioned muscle mass, what will result is the skin and weak muscles.

Professional advice: To minimize the loss of valuable muscle mass and damage to your metabolism, I recommend that you strive for a gradual decrease in weight. 1-2 pounds a month is a healthy benchmark to look for.

By setting too much a goal at the beginning, you often venture out of failure because of the lack of knowledge and motivation to achieve it, as well as the disappointment that may occur when you see the first undesirable visual effects of a possible rapid weight loss.

Once I recommend a weight loss within these limits, I often get the answer, "Is not that too small?"

It is not too much considering the length of time that action has been taken - this is the main mistake rather than the "slow weight loss". If you lose 2 pounds a week, you will lose over 15 pounds in 2 months, but you will have a tremendous chance of keeping them.

In Brief: High intake of protein will help maintain valuable muscle mass that gives a tight and beautiful look to the body.

It will also help keep your metabolism high, especially when combined with strength training. This way you make sure that what is below the fat will actually look good.

What is the optimal intake of protein?

It has been shown that the optimal amount of protein depends on many individual factors. Some of them include physical activity, age, muscle mass, fitness goals, health, and more.

Then what amount of protein is best suited to weight loss, muscle gain or health improvement?

There is no universal rule for determining individual protein needs for which there is complete consensus.

Rather, "norms of sufficiency" are adopted for non-sponsoring people.

However, sportspeople are always looking for maximum recovery and development, so they need more accurate norms. Which is the right approach?

You may have paid attention to the recommended daily food consumption labels - ~ 56 grams per day for men and ~ 46 grams for women.

The bottom line for these recommendations is that they are based on an average man or woman who receives 2000 calories a day.

Age, specific daily activities, calories, energy consumption, and other factors are not considered.

This amount may be enough to prevent a serious deficiency but is far from optimal for weight loss, muscle gain or good health.

Optimum reception for unsporting

For children: Between 34 and 52 g of protein per day.

For adult men and women: Between 0.8 and 1 g protein per kilogram or 25-30% of the total calorie intake of the day.

Optimal reception for sportsmen

For amateurs and sports lovers: Between 1.5 and 2.2 grams of protein per kilogram a day.

For professionals and advanced trainees: Between 2 and 3 grams of protein per kilogram per day.

To calculate an estimate of how much protein a sport lover needs, we can use the following calculation: 80 (kilograms) x 2.2 (grams of protein) = 176 grams of protein per day.

Professional advice: Choose a higher protein intake limit to make sure you meet your needs and give the body the needed restoration and development. Rarely can be overpowered by taking protein in good health.

In short: Recommended daily doses of protein are very different for sports and non-sportsmen. Sports enthusiasts and more advanced trainees need a higher protein intake every day - between 1.5 and 3 grams of protein per kilogram.

When to take protein?

The most optimal option is to distribute protein throughout the day by eating protein with each meal.

Once you've determined optimal protein intake, you can divide the result from the number of meals per day.

Example: We calculated the need for a sports enthusiast who is 80 pounds. In his diet there are 4 meals a day. Divide the required protein daily (176 grams) into the number of meals (4 meals). The calculation looks like this: 176 (grams of protein per day) / 4 (meals per day) = ~ 44 g of protein at each meal.

Professional advice: Be sure to add protein to your breakfast. A common mistake is the lack of valuable proteins early in the morning. Taking protein in combination with other foods will help you start your day in the best way. Examples of sources of protein that you can include at breakfast are eggs, skimmed cottage cheese, powdered protein, and more.

In short: The best option is to take protein to each meal in even portions. If you've calculated that you need 200 grams of protein and you consume 3 meals a day, you need ~ 66 grams of protein at each meal.

How to Get More Protein In The Diet?

Increasing intake of protein in the diet is simple, but it often takes time to prepare.

This is also the main reason most people do not base their meals on a protein basis but on carbohydrates and fats.

Another reason is the price of quality protein sources that do not contain high amounts of saturated fat.

However, there are variants that are easy to prepare, available as a price and do not contain a large number of calories.

Animal Foods:

• Meat and meat products - chicken, veal, pork

• Eggs

• Fish and seafood

•Milk and milk products

Plant sources:

•Bean cultures

• Nuts

• Cereals

•Seeds

Virtually any natural food contains a certain percentage of protein in its composition. However, the greatest contribution to the provision of amino acids to the body has food containing at least 7 percent or more of protein in its composition.

Foods with 3-7% content have a minor role.

Each food in the groups listed has its own nutritional value, which, besides its protein content, is determined by a number of other factors: amino acid profile, biological value, rate of absorption, and others.

The question is, "Which food is the best choice among foods rich in protein?" The answer is, "There is no absolute champion!" The reason for this is that different proteins supply the body with different amounts and proportions of amino acids within a different period of time after consumption.

The best approach is the varied diet - the alternation of different quality sources of protein.

Animal protein sources are believed to outperform the plant at a direct comparison of the amino acid gram profile per gram due to the increased presence of essential amino acids in the animal protein composition.

This is even more important for sports people who have increased needs for these amino acids.

Professional advice: If you are on a low carb diet, you can afford more calorie sources of protein (with more fat). If you do not adhere to a low carbohydrate diet, you should try to maximize fat-free protein sources.

This rule will allow you to maintain higher protein intake without taking too many calories.

In short: Every natural food contains a quantity of protein, but there are ones that provide more than others. Animal protein sources are believed to outperform the plant by the diversity and saturation of valuable amino acids (important for sportsmen).

When it comes to fat loss and good-looking body, protein is the king of nutrients.

You do not have to make serious restrictions to take advantage of higher protein intake.

This is especially appealing to many who want to lose weight because most high-protein foods are also delicious.

High protein diet can be an effective long-term strategy to prevent obesity and maintain a good physical form, not just a remedy to use from time to time to lose fat.

By increasing protein intake, you will balance the "calories and calories burned" equation to your advantage.

So, for months, years, or decades, the waist difference can be enormous without much effort in dieting.

Despite the benefits of weight loss, such as appetite reduction and increased metabolism, you should keep in mind that you will not lose significant weight unless you consume less calories than you take. One gram of protein contains 4 calories and they are added to the total daily energy intake.

You may be quite pleasantly surprised by the amount of food you can eat with a high protein diet, especially if you are currently eating mostly unhealthy food while at the same time you will reach a calorie deficit.

7 Effective ways to control the appetite for sweet and unhealthy foods

Do you often have the desire for sweet and other unhealthy foods that you try to avoid at all costs but cannot control your appetite?

Hunger for certain foods and resisting temptation can be a real challenge, especially when we allow our energy levels to run out over a longer period of time.

That's why the body is powered by the right fuel to help solve the problem.

The tips of the article share with my clients about their diet. To motivate yourself to apply what you read, I present feedback from them:

• "I did not expect a moment to eat junk and junk." - YH;

• "For the first time I have a week without eating jam and eating food. Now I have the feeling that I can enjoy them when I think and the feeling is great "- C.L.

Consuming your favourite foods, though unhealthy, would not hurt so much, even if you follow a weight loss plan.

As long as this is consistent with other parameters of your diet and is not a constant phenomenon in uncontrolled quantities, because you will do your efforts to fail.

Here are 7 effective ways to help you control the desire for sweet and unhealthy foods.

It is important to remember that this type of physiological hunger for certain foods usually happens for some reason. This article will guide you and what to follow.

Composition of Meals

The composition of your meals can greatly help to reduce your appetite.

When done properly, you will allow your body to control your blood sugar levels much more effectively.

Excluding a large group of foods that supply a variety of nutrients is one way to ensure uncontrollable appetite and constant hunger, especially if you have no dietary experience behind you.

Protein sources (meat and eggs fillet), healthy fats (raw nuts, olive oil), low glycemic index carbohydrates (brown rice, oatmeal), vegetables and 1-2 fruits will help effectively regulate blood sugar levels in day-to-day and are one of the strongest weapons to tackle the problem.

The lack of vegetables in your daily meals is one of the most serious mistakes. They can satiate you for a long time in combination with other foods but without providing extra calories. The only minus will come from this if you taste them with unspoilt amounts of salt and fat.

Hydration

Maintaining good hydration is essential to control appetite.

If you are dehydrated, it is very likely to create an imbalance in the levels of sodium in the body. This in turn leads to a desire to eat foods rich in salt, which are often unhealthy and many calories.

How do you know how much water you need?

Although the answer varies with personal weight, age, physical activity, and a number of other factors, a good example would be: If you weigh 70 pounds, a healthy amount of water would be between 2.5 - 4 litres of water per day. When determining what limit to choose, consider: climate, physical activity and sweating.

Frequency of Meals

Numerous studies have shown that eating does not directly affect body temperature, heart rhythm, and changes in blood tests that lead to the loss of excess fat and kilos as it has been thought for a long time.

But in the same study, it was claimed that people who had been given only 1 meal a day had a much greater degree of hunger.

Following a plan that distributes your calorie intake evenly throughout the day will allow you to regulate your appetite by maintaining more stable blood sugar levels.

The feeling that you always have available food and are charged with energy acts positively on the psyche and can further help.

In combination with the above tips, you will be one more step closer to the desired goals.

Replace your favourite foods with healthier versions

Replacing foods that you find it hard to quit is a good approach that can save too many calories. Example replacements you can make:

1. Cold yogurt with fresh fruit instead of ice cream;

2. Slices of carrots and cucumber with humus instead of chips;

3. Dark Chocolate instead of Milk Chocolate;

4. Homemade roasted popcorn instead of a large quantity of fat;

5. Whole wheat bread or sliced peanut butter instead of donut;

6. Shredded meat for minced meat instead of minced meat with added lard, salt, preservatives, etc .;

7. A healthier version of pizza cooked home with wholemeal or cauliflower instead of bought;

8. Whole-grained spaghetti or pasta with homemade sauce prepared from vegetables instead of ready-made or from restaurant;

9. Coffee sweetened with a natural sweetener instead of coffee with sugar or honey and cream.

Preparation of food and flavouring

Time separation in preparing and flavouring food is also important.

Different cooking styles can diversify your meals. The use of natural spices such as black pepper, red pepper, marjoram, thyme, savoury, natural apple vinegar, freshly squeezed lemon juice, etc. is highly recommended.

Cinnamon, fenugreek, linseed, and skimmed cottage cheese are foods that are known to suppress appetite. Good practice would be to consume them before your favourite calorie options.

Combining everything written will help satisfy your gustatory needs and will be another step towards regulating your uncontrollable appetite.

Quality sleep

The link between lack of quality sleep and low levels of the hormone leptin - a hormone that controls appetite, has been proven, while the levels of the hormone responsible for the stimulation of hunger - ghirlin are rising.

Not surprisingly, people with poor sleep usually have problems with their eating habits.

7-8 hours of sleep within 24 hours can significantly affect your appetite control throughout the day.

Breakfast

Skipping breakfast, as well as choosing the wrong one, is a prerequisite for many to confuse your whole day.

Starting the day with a healthy breakfast containing essential nutrients is a perfect way to lay the foundation for the upcoming day.

You may feel that coffee or juice is enough to start your day full, but they are not able to fuel the body with fuel for a longer period of time.

This is very likely, very soon after the breakfast in question, to reach out to what is most affordable and convenient to eat, namely fast and unhealthy food.

On the other hand, if you are feeding your body in full, you will be less likely to feel a great appetite or hunger for the next few hours.

How would a healthy breakfast look like to give energy for hours ahead?

Option 1: Whole eggs (source of high-quality protein and useful fat), combined with oatmeal (source of mainly complex carbohydrates), combined and cooked according to personal preference.

Option 2: Whey protein powder (mainly source of high-quality protein), combined with raw nuts (mainly derived from useful fats) and oatmeal combined according to taste and purpose.

The Most Popular Weight Loss Diets: Pros and Cons (+ How to Choose the Most Suitable for You)

When it comes to weight loss, you may experience over 100 different diets and ways that promise fast weight loss.

Magazines, books and websites claim to have found the key to weight reduction - from diets that limit fat or carbohydrates to those who offer super foods or special supplements to achieve the desired appearance.

With so many different and often contradictory opinions and weight loss tips, it is extremely difficult to make the right choice.

This article will introduce you to some of the most popular diets as well as their pros and cons to choose the safest and most effective option tailored to your individual needs and goals to achieve the results you've always wanted.

- 1 # 1. Low fat diet

- 2 # 2. Vegan or Vegetarian diet

- 3 # 3. Mediterranean diet

- 4 # 4. Paleo diet

- 5 # 5: Separate Feeding

- 6 # 6: Individual Program

- 7 # 7: Conclusion

1. Low fat diet

This type of diet does not focus on calories or carbohydrates, but on limiting fat intake.

Diet that totally limits fat can be dangerous as they are the source of the important fatty acids the body needs to function properly.

Pros: Fats contain 9 calories per gram, and carbohydrates and proteins - 4 calories per gram.

This way you can reduce the total number of calories and achieve weight loss.

Cons: Fats are necessary for the human body to function properly.

They can help regulate appetite, healthy hormonal changes and feed the body with valuable nutrients.

The complete restriction over a longer period of time can cause serious damage to metabolism and hormones.

Common delusions: Many foods and drinks are promoted as low-fat ones. Often, if such food is delicious, it is reworked to reduce calories, but artificial improvers are added that are extremely harmful to health.

An example is a non-fat yogurt but with added sugar or glucose-fructose syrup.

Another popular fallacy is that body fat is being fat-fed. The truth is that we will gain fat when we take a lot more calories than we burn, rather than choosing a source of calories in our menu.

For whom it is appropriate: Suitable for people who exercise actively and can burn the energy that carbs provide.

In this way, physical activity will burn up accumulated stocks, and limiting calories from reducing fat intake will help for faster weight reduction.

2. Vegan or Vegetarian Diet

The vegetarian diet excludes meat consumption. In the vegan, besides meat, no animal products are consumed - egg, milk, fish, etc.

This diet is usually low-calorie, low-fat and rich in vitamins and minerals.

Pros: This type of diets are usually low-calorie.

They can help lower cholesterol and blood pressure.

Most vegetarians consume a lot of vegetables and fruits, something that is often overlooked in the modern menu.

Loss can be achieved in kilograms without excluding favorite foods, as calorie intake is usually very limited.

Cons: The animal products contain important nutrients that do not abound in plant sources.

A common deficiency seen in vegans and vegetarians is group B vitamins.

Also in reducing animal feed, it is difficult to obtain proteins with a full amino acid profile (high values of all body building blocks).

This may adversely affect the athletes who aim to increase muscle mass, shape and tighten the body.

Common delusions: Absolutely all nutrients can be obtained without consuming animal products.

While in theory this may be so, in practice, many people have neither the knowledge nor the discipline to do so.

For this reason, this type of diet is extremely inappropriate for adolescents, pregnant, lactating, elderly, and people recovering from injuries or injuries.

For whom it is appropriate: It may be appropriate for overweight people, cholesterol and blood pressure control, and for people who do not want to consume meat for personal convictions.

3. The Mediterranean diet

The diet is based on fresh and simple foods.

It is based on the food consumed by people from Italy and Greece. They are known to consume lots of vegetables and fruits, olive oil, unprocessed dairy products, nuts and fish.

The diet is popular because of extremely low levels of heart disease, cancer, diabetes and obesity in these regions.

Pros: The biggest benefits are that there is no complete restriction in any group of foods, but the processed ones are not to be honoured.

It can have a favourable effect on maintaining and improving health.

Cons: Serious weight loss cannot be expected.

The positive effects of the diet will be healthier rather than visual.

Greater budget is needed than other type of diet or diet.

Frequent delusions: It is a common delusion that food and beverages can be consumed in unlimited quantities as long as they are healthy, vegan or bio.

While a handful of raw nuts are extremely beneficial to health and will deliver valuable and diverse nutrients, it should be borne in mind that 100 grams of raw almonds contain almost 600 calories.

It is extremely easy to overeat the amount of food that is associated with the Mediterranean diet and make it impossible to lose weight.

Who it is for: Try this diet if you want to improve your health, but you do not need a big weight loss.

It will be easier to follow this regime if you like the idea of eating mainly foods and beverages in their natural form (closest to nature).

4. Paleo diet

The diet is related to the ancient man's diet - mainly meat, fish, fruits, vegetables, nuts and eggs.

This type of diet completely excludes man-made foods and dairy products.

Pros: The Paleo diet will significantly reduce blood sugar levels and regulate insulin sensitivity - extremely beneficial to health.

It can lead to serious weight loss due to the restriction of the intake of processed foods, which are often calorie.

Cons: To achieve long-term results with diet or diet, it is necessary to introduce changes in your lifestyle that can last over time.

The Paleo diet completely restricts the foods that the modern man has become accustomed to, and is constantly surrounded - such as dairy products, processed foods, flavoured drinks, and more.

This is a serious prerequisite for failure or recovery of old kilos after the regime has ended.

It can be extremely difficult to follow the palate diet if you can not cook for yourself or eat often outside.

Frequent delusions: As with the Mediterranean diet, here is also considered that there is no need to limit the quantities, as dietary choices are entirely in the box healthy.

Although a food is healthy or not, it contains calories. If we take more calories than we burn, we will not be able to achieve serious weight loss.

The diet consumes larger amounts of meat, fish and eggs, and it misleads some that it is not necessary to eat vegetables and fruits.

To whom it is appropriate: Try this diet if you are highly motivated to achieve results and have serious discipline in the kitchen.

Do not pick up the palate diet if you have no dietary experience, and if you have no energy and desire to cook yourself.

The diet is also not suitable for those who cannot imagine life without jam.

5. Separate Feeding

Separate nutrition is a nutrition system that considers food as a pool of nutrients divided into several clearly defined groups.

The aim is to define a methodology for their effective combining to improve digestion, reduce digestion and digestion time, and reduce digestive tract products.

The most popular diets for weight loss in Bulgaria are based on the principle of the separate diet, namely "90-day diet"

Pros: Separated nutrition is believed to help facilitate the absorption of nutrients from the body and facilitate its work to achieve weight loss.

Because of the limitation of certain dietary sources on different days, the total number of calories is extremely low compared to what people are not accustomed to eating.

The total number of calories taken is the most important prerequisite for weight loss and weight reduction.

For this reason, first results can be seen very quickly, as well as achieving weight reduction without achieving a standstill over a longer period of time compared to other regimens.

Cons: Stretch marks, cellulite and yo-yo effects are often accompanying side effects due to the amount of muscle mass that is lost by aggressive reduction in calorie intake.

Several days in Ninety-Day Diet is based on carbohydrate sources - simple and complex. Frequent intake of this type of food source can lead to permanent insulin secretion, a serious prerequisite for fat burning, and the development of diabetes.

Another big downside of restrictive diets is that this type of diet can slow your metabolism (metabolism) and even damage it long term.

Much of these inconveniences can be reduced if the separate diet is combined with exercise.

Common delusions: Many people believe that in order to achieve a beautiful and harmonious body, it is necessary to simply lose weight.

This is extremely false, and many of those who have passed the 90-day diet say they feel cheated by what regimes offer.

The reason is that most people who undergo these restrictive diets are those who want extremely fast results and are often unwilling to make extra efforts by doing sports.

To whom it is appropriate: For people who want to achieve rapid weight loss, even if it is at the expense of health.

Extremely unsuitable for adolescents, pregnant, lactating, elderly, and people recovering from injuries or injuries.

6. Individual program

Sample Diet and Training Program

If you have tried different diets but unsuccessfully, you have probably come to the conclusion that everyone is missing something extremely important for it to be successful.

This is the individual approach that is needed to achieve and retain results.

The reason? Every organism is different. It is not possible for a diet to be suitable for a person weighing 70 pounds and one who weighs 110 pounds.

Pros: Everything in the diet is made especially for you.

Meals are tailored to your experience with diets, budget, food and drink preferences, allergies, and more.

If you can stick to a certain amount of time (usually about a month), there is no way you cannot get serious results.

In addition, you get constant support, which is often the missing link for achieving and retaining results.

Cons: Although food and beverages are tailored to personal preferences, in order to achieve results, it may be necessary to compromise on the menu on both sides.

It should also be borne in mind that such an approach may not be attractive to anyone in financial terms.

In order to achieve a serious result, you must be prepared to follow specific guidelines, trusting one person at large.

Frequent delusions: The mistakes associated with such type of individual services are not very much, as with professional information, almost all parameters are clear in advance.

However, a popular fallacy is that one and the same food should be consumed throughout the program.

Who it is for: For people who do not want to waste time on samples and mistakes.

Try different diets without success.

For people who are charged with energy by others and want to follow specific guidelines.

For those who want to achieve a reasonable weight change, but at the same time improve their health and the way they look.

If you want to follow your own diet and cooking, this program may not be right for you.

7. Conclusion

As a conclusion, I will add a few tips that will increase your chances of achieving desired results many times.

Tip # 1 for Success with Diet: Avoid too restrictive diets

Restrictive diets are regimens that promise to help you lose weight quickly, but as mentioned, they are always associated with unwanted side effects.

Such diets often cause starvation, which can be dangerous for metabolism, hormones and overall health.

Recovering from this type of diet can take months, and continue with unhealthy eating habits and low physical activity, even years.

Tip # 2 for diet success: Stick to unprocessed and healthy foods

Whichever diet you choose, stick to the foods that are closest to your natural state - with minimal human handling. The fewer the processes you pass the food you eat, the more intact will be its beneficial nutrients.

Minus here is that healthy and unprofitable choices are often more expensive than the most used products on the market.

To make this step more accessible, you might want to consider buying your food as a bulk, as well as shopping from private farmers or markets.

Tip # 3 for Diet Success: Combine with Exercise

Each diet can be supplemented by exercises - cardio activity, weight training or both.

Combining cardio workout and weight training is the best possible option from a healthy perspective as well as achieving quick and effective results.

Any extra activity will help when your primary goal is weight loss.

Even a walk in the park will have health benefits.

It is recommended ~ 150 minutes of weekly physical activity to maintain good health and ~ 300 minutes per week to achieve healthy weight loss.

Tip # 4 for Success with a Diet: Find support from a friend

No matter what diet you choose, possibly do it with a friend.

Someone who can hold you accountable may be everything you need to succeed.

This can be a friend you think you have a right nutrition or a family member to support you in difficult moments.

If you do not have such a contact, it is best to contact a qualified fitness instructor.

This advice is valid with double strength if you are pregnant, nursing, teenage, adult, or have any health problems.

The last thing you want is your diet to cause health problems.

It is therefore highly advisable to consult with a specialist, even if you have already chosen an action plan. Everybody is different, and the diet you choose may not be appropriate for yours.

Easy Ways to Weight Loss Without Diet

To lose weight and lose weight, it is necessary to burn more calories than we consume, which means one: control of the portions.

But this does not necessarily mean that this process must be linked to hunger until it reaches the desired outcomes, as it is perceived by popular unhealthy diets.

There is a much easier way to lose weight and keep the results.

Weight Loss Without Diet - How Does It Work?

The easiest way to lose weight and retention of results is actually by introducing healthy replacements.

The main reasons why this method is extremely effective are 3:

Reason # 1: You will be able to limit your calorie intake

Limiting calories intake without hunger.

This is possible due to the fact that unprocessed foods (often categorized as healthy) are usually more bulky than processed ones.

The better news is that you do not have to completely unhook unhealthy food from the menu. Favourite ice cream, chocolate, chips and others can be part of a healthy menu, but not its basis.

Imagine how much food you can consume for the same or fewer calories, leading to the next point:

Reason # 2: You will regulate appetite and feelings of hunger

Choosing healthier choices throughout the day will take a variety of nutrients and give your body what it needs.

Larger portions will allow you to feel fuller for a longer time and do not feel the need for harmful food.

A basic rule I recommend to follow:

When you feel the need for unhealthy food, first eat a balanced, healthy diet containing a variety of macro and micronutrients - proteins, carbohydrates, beneficial fats, vitamins and minerals.

You will be convinced that by leaving unhealthy foods for the last time, you will often have no need of them or it will be so small that you will be able to control it with ease.

Reason # 3: You will adjust blood sugar and insulin sensitivity

Most processed foods classified as "harmful food" have a man-made composition.

This change most often removes a useful part of a particular product to make it look better, more delicious, with a smoother smell or, in other words, give it a commercial look.

However, this affects the composition of the product, most often making it poorer to nutrients.

The poorer is a food of a variety of macro elements (proteins, carbohydrates, fats, fibre), the greater the unhealthy rise in blood sugar will cause.

These upsets are associated with an energy flow that is available for a very short period of time - a few minutes.

The problem is that in a few minutes we cannot burn calories from a cake that has given us 1000+ calories.

The body will use what it needs - whether the source is healthy or unhealthy, but what it does not need will store as fat.

Besides the negative influence on weight and weight, frequent increases and decreases in blood sugar are associated with the development of type 2 diabetes.

The best you can do for yourself is to consume more unprocessed and less processed foods.

A great list of suggestions on healthy options will be read in the article below.

Why should not we limit calories when we aim at weight loss.

Since the most important rule of weight loss is the number of calories you receive, I also think the following question: Why do not we just limit calories to the minimum to create the deficit and thus lose weight quickly?

The reason is that our bodies are adapted to adapt to any external and internal effects for self-preservation.

In order for the body to function properly and at high revs, it needs to be powered.

Lower calorie intake is associated with deficits that are harmful not only to health but also to maintaining optimal weight.

When receiving a low calorie count, the body:

• Losing muscle mass that tightens and gives a beautiful look;

• Goes into Sleep Mode, which means you will burn less calories, no matter how small you take or how much you sport;

• Such type of restrictions are associated with weight loss, but are often accompanied by stretch marks, cellulite and loose skin.

What healthy replacements do we apply?

I'm introducing easy ways to reduce your portions, reduce your calories and lose fat - without counting your minutes to your next meal.

Healthy Replacement # 1: Water instead of other beverages

Drink 300-500 ml. water before meals.

Filling your stomach with water will make you naturally reduce your intake of food afterwards.

You will also reduce the intake of other beverages that are often unhealthy and add extra calories to your menu.

It is scientifically proven that our brain confuses signals of hunger and dehydration - we may often feel a great need for food without hunger if we take too little water every day. Another reason to consume more water.

If drinking water is too boring or difficult to do, just add natural ingredients to it. Several healthy suggestions are:

No calories and sugar: lemon, lime, cucumber, mint stalk, ginger, natural cinnamon, natural apple vinegar, rosemary, thyme and others.

With a minimal amount of calories and sugar: strawberries, blueberries, kiwi and more.

According to your personal goals, you can diversify the ingredients you use and test different combinations.

If you have difficulty reducing drinks you are accustomed to, you can start with smaller steps. A good example is by replacing carbonated beverages and natural juices with freshly squeezed fruits such as grapefruit, kiwi and orange.

Healthy Replacement # 2: Vegetables instead of calorie foods

Adding vegetables to each meal is a sure way to reduce your calorie intake and eat less unhealthy foods.

Vegetables are a source of valuable nutrients like vitamins, minerals and fibre.

Consuming more vegetables will reduce the natural intake of foods high in calories.

Healthy Change # 3: Healthy Breakfast Instead of Fast Food

Starting the day with a full meal is a good prerequisite for keeping healthy eating habits throughout the day.

To reduce your intake of calories in breakfast, you can replace some of the most used ingredients with their less calorie and healthier alternatives.

Similar examples are:

• Replacement of whole milk with low fat;

• Replacement of muesli and cereal mixes with oatmeal with fresh fruit;

• Replace sugar with honey and cinnamon, and as a next step, replace honey with stevia and cinnamon;

• Replace carbonated beverages or natural juice with freshly squeezed juice or water.

Healthy Replacement # 4: Cooking at Home instead of eating outdoors

Even if you try to eat healthy in a restaurant, there are things that are completely out of your control.

An example is the flavour of even vegetables with calorie supplements, as well as added fat to dishes that at first seem healthy.

The preparation of food at home allows better monitoring of the amounts and calories received, as well as a better selection of products.

It also ensures that no poor food is consumed or consumed, which is also a basic prerequisite for diet failure.

Healthy Replace # 5: Whole Fruit instead of Purchased Natural Juice

Natural juice, which is widespread and accepted as healthy, does not actually contain cellulose and skin from the fruit, which significantly reduces the amount of valuable nutrients, such as fibre.

In addition, artificial amounts of sugar and / or glucose-fructose syrup are often added to it.

For this reason, to get the full health benefits of the fruit, choose a whole fruit instead of a natural fruit juice.

Healthy replacement # 6: Local produce instead of import

If you can, choose products that are produced near you.

A number of studies have shown that local fruits and vegetables that are in season can be much more nutritious.

Or paraphrased: It is much more useful to eat seasonal fruits and vegetables such as apples and tomatoes than bananas and mangoes.

Healthy Replacement # 7: Butter and balsamic vinegar instead of processed ready-made dressing

You've probably been paying attention to the large number of ingredients that contain the various options of ready-made dressing, as well as the large number of calories from unhealthy sources.

With such a flavour we turn a healthy and useful food into extremely unhealthy.

A better option would be to make your own dressing with olive oil, balsamic vinegar, lemon or lime, etc.

Or get closer to ready-made dresses with a similar number of ingredients, but from good sources.

Healthy replacement # 10: Fresh fruit instead of syrup

Flavour extra pancakes or other fresh fruit instead of syrup, jam, honey and more.

This will not only significantly reduce calories from unhealthy sources, but will also provide you with an energy supply without adversely affecting your blood sugar.

Healthy Replacement # 8: Pure alcohol instead of cocktails and impurities

When consuming alcohol, choose cleaner options that contain a minimum of ingredients and no added sugar.

Similar examples are red wine and vodka instead of cocktails that can reach up to 1000 calories per serving.

Healthy Replacement # 9: Brown rice instead of white rice

Although white rice has its benefits, especially for fitness purposes, for most people who aim at weight loss, brown rice is a better option.

The reason is that it does not remove the outer shell containing beneficial nutrients such as fibre.

Healthy Replacement # 10: Whole Grains instead of Processed

Whole wheat bread and pasta from whole wheat contains valuable nutrients such as antioxidants and fibre.

Much more appropriate choices to their revised versions - white bread, pasta, spaghetti, etc., when we aim at weight loss and weight reduction.

Healthy Replacement # 11: Oatmeal instead of muesli

Choose oatmeal instead of muesli and breakfast cereals.

If necessary, flavour with cinnamon, stew, fruit or honey.

Oatmeal is sometimes better than all marketplaces. In the second option, besides the natural sugar from the fruits, 90% of the cases add extra to improve the taste.

Healthy replacement # 12: 3 meals a day instead of omitting meals

Eat a main meal at least 3 times a day instead of skipping meals.

When you do not take the time to make a healthy meal, you will often find yourself in a situation where you are forced to resort to a food or drink that you know will harm your regime and move you away from the goal.

Taking main meals at regular intervals throughout the day will ensure that you have the energy and tone to perform your everyday tasks in the most effective way.

At the same time, you will get weight loss and weight reduction by making healthier choices and taking fewer calories.

Healthy Replacement # 13: Natural mustard instead of mayonnaise

Mustard is a kind of spice, which is mainly put on sandwiches and salads. The main ingredients in it are the seeds of the mustard plant. When making the seeds, they are ground into powder and vinegar, salt, water and oil are added.

A much healthier and less calorie alternative to mayonnaise.

Keep in mind that mustard is a hot spice and can cause an allergic reaction if you are prone.

Healthy Replacement # 14: Avocado instead of butter

Make avocado puree and use it for garnish, grease or even cooking.

Wholegrain bread can add avocado, tomato and sea or Himalayan salt for delicious and healthy intermediate meals.

Healthy Replacement # 15: Clean meats instead of sausages

Choose meat that is clean and free of additives or with minimal added ingredients.

Often, salt, preservatives, bacon and other unnecessary ingredients are added to minced meat or popular ready-made products, which not only adds a lot of calories to your menu but is also dangerous to health.

Under pure meats are meant chicken and turkey fillets, white fish, calf carcass, pork schnitzel and counter fillet and similar variants.

Note that as a healthy replacement I do not recommend clean meats instead of those with higher% fat as they can also have a place in a well-balanced diet.

Healthy Replacement # 16: Home Food instead of Overeating

I have often come across situations where food is eating at the table, only to keep it.

When we pursue fitness goals and want to work on reducing the waist centimetres, it is a must to not overeat.

A much better option would be to take your food home and consume it a little later.

Try the 80/20 rule.

It consists of stopping eating once you feel that you are a total of 80%. If you do not have self-control, just serve 20% less food than you are accustomed to.

Healthy Replacement # 17: Slow chewing instead of fast food

Maintaining a healthy weight does not include just what we eat. Studies show that how we eat is also of great importance.

A university study proves that people who eat their food more slowly consume less total calories.

The science behind this: Our bodies need time to feel satiety. For this reason, the slower we chew, the more time we give the brain to register satiety signals.

Another thing you can get from this study is that the type of food you consume also has a serious impact.

Participants in the study, who consumed cereals and whole grains, received significantly fewer calories than those who consumed refined options such as white bread and roasted and salted products.

Scientists give much of the health benefits of fibre contained in unprocessed foods.

The conclusion that can be made is that choosing healthy choices - unprocessed foods is key to achieving weight loss without diet.

Healthy Replacement # 18: Black coffee instead of flavoured coffee

When you combine coffee with cream and sugar, the calories you add to your menu will have a major impact.

In addition to additional excess calories, sugar gives quick energy that affects insulin.

On the other hand, pure coffee can help you lose weight faster and reduce excess pounds.

Caffeine is actually a commonly used ingredient in the most effective fat burning and weight loss supplements.

If you need to taste your coffee, use the tips of point # 9.

Healthy Replacement # 19: Whole-grained homemade sandwich instead of toaster

A toaster can provide a huge amount of calories from unhealthy sources, especially if you use the most commonly offered garnish - fried potatoes (semi-baked) and sauces.

A much healthier choice to control your calorie intake would be to make a whole-wheat bread sandwich by adding ham, cooked potatoes, tomato, avocado, spices, and more.

Healthy replacement # 20: Cooked eggs instead of fried

Eggs and oatmeal is one of the best snacks you can make. The combination provides absolutely everything for a complete start of the day our bodies need.

Keep in mind that slightly boiled eggs (loaves) retain much of their beneficial nutrients.

While a large amount of protein is found in the protein, most of the vitamins and minerals are actually concentrated in yolk.

For this reason, I do not recommend that you fall into extremes and discard all yolks.

2-3 yolk a day would not harm anything but would provide beneficial fat, protein and a full range of vitamins and minerals.

Healthy Replacement # 21: Raw nuts instead of nut oil

Nuts often add refined olive oil, sugar and other ingredients that do not have any benefit in a weight loss diet.

It is also much easier to take large amounts of peanut and almond oil calories, compared to their equivalent in raw nuts.

The next few examples are not food-related but most of them have a proven positive effect when we're aiming at reducing calories and losing weight.

Healthy Replacement # 22: Dream instead of an energy drink

When you feel the need for energy, instead of consuming an energy drink, choose to sleep.

Sleep deficiency increases hunger and has a negative effect on metabolism.

This is related to the level of cortisol (the stress hormone), which can rise even when you are sitting.

Sleeping over eight o'clock in the morning would also give you more energy during the day and increase levels of growth hormone that is involved directly in burning fat and regulating other important hormones.

Also, most energy drinks contain a large amount of sugar (30-50 grams per pack), and their alternatives with 0 calories - a large number of chemical ingredients that are proven to be harmful to health.

Healthy Replacement # 23: Healthy Food Instead of Junk Food

Easy-to-use advice that can reduce the consumption of unwanted foods and beverages is simply not to buy while shopping.

This way you will not have convenient and quick access to them.

So when it comes to eating, the chance to get better food is multiplied.

Healthy Replacement # 24: Shopping City instead of fasting

Several studies have shown that people who go shopping fast-food buy more than 40% more products that they realize is harmful to them.

Healthy Replacement # 25: Average Plate instead of Large

Smaller plates can save you over 20% of the calories you would have consumed on a larger plate.

Healthy Replacement # 26: Eat on a table instead in front of a TV

Eat at a table designed for this purpose. Feeding in front of the TV can lead to serious overeating and unhealthy selection of products.

TV viewers are more likely to be distracted and lose track of the amounts consumed, and this easily leads to overeating.

There are studies that prove that television (sound and picture) can interfere with internal signs (real feelings of hunger or satiety) and this again has a serious negative effect.

There is also a much higher chance of choosing unhealthy snack while watching TV.

Healthy Replacement # 27: Sticks instead of fork

Interesting advice I came across in several weight loss materials.

The recommendation here is to try to eat with sticks instead of a fork.

For some it can be a challenge, but certainly this technique will help slower and more meaningful nutrition.

Healthy Replacement # 28: Teeth wash instead of chewing gum

Tooth brushing results in a sense of cleanliness and freshness. This will keep you longer without putting anything in your mouth.

Keep in mind that juices and acids are released when chewing.

These reactions give the body signals to trigger the digestive system and this may adversely affect blood sugar and insulin.

For this reason, you will also not allow your gastrointestinal tract to relax if you chew gums frequently.

All chewing gums contain at least 1 of the ingredients, but most often in the composition are combinations of: colorants and other compounds for a better commercial appearance, sugar or aspartame for a better taste.

Healthy Replacement # 29: Fitness or Yoga instead of Stress

Stress may slow your metabolism. The hormone released in stressful situations - cortisol, prevents the body from burning fat. So try to include even a minimal amount of movement or sport.

Dirty Eating: How to use it to improve our diet

How do we use dirty meals to stick to our diet - without getting fat and at the same time getting extra benefits from them?

Dirty meals can improve the way you look, control your appetite during a diet, and help to lose excess fat.

Once you've chosen a diet or diet that's right for you, the question remains - how to include all the favourite foods that you suppose you do not have to consume without compromising your results.

Some choose the ultimate approach, limiting all harmful foods to 100%, driven by the desire to achieve faster results.

The problem is that this approach is most often chosen by people without much dietary experience.

Without having pre-established eating habits and experience to allow for flexibility in the diet, it is very difficult to keep this type of regime for a long time in order to achieve desired goals and to keep the results achieved.

From a hormonal and psychological point of view it is considered a good idea to have a favourite but "unhealthy food" in the regime. This approach is known as the rule or principle 90/10.

The rule is a diet in which 90% of calories come from healthy foods and the other 10% of favourite foods and beverages.

These 10% can be 1-2 meals per week of pizza, ice cream, spaghetti with sauce, black chocolate and more.

Depending on your goals and current status, you can use dirty food as a plus.

For example, if you want to remove excess fat, it would be better to choose a nutrition chew to give you pleasure but at the same time to have a high nutritional value. Examples are black chocolate and spaghetti.

While muscle mass growth is a priority but not a lower% fat, then it would be acceptable to choose ice cream, sweets and others like dirty meals.

Common mistakes associated with eating dirty meals

Mistake # 1: Dirty day instead of dirty food

Turning a single dirty meal into eating inappropriate meals throughout the day is common.

One reason is that people do not stop for a second to think about how much additional unnecessary calories they can take for an all-day indiscriminate meal.

The other thing is that a dirty meal can confuse the created routine or diet, and then all the other meals of the day go wrong.

Emotional eating is the third reason. Not everyone can control and return to their regime after the planned dirty meal.

This is not only detrimental to the physics you seek for stomach health, but it also creates a link with food, which can be a serious obstacle to achieving long-term results.

Mistake# 2: No Preliminary Plan

If you do not have planned dirty meals on a particular day, there is a great chance you can do more than you need.

For example, you're having a pizza on Thursday, and on Friday you know you're on a birthday.

To make sure you do not go over dirty meals, it's a good idea to determine exactly what day they are going to be.

Of course, this day may suffer changes if necessary, but the most optimal fitness goals are dirty meals to be around a heavy workout or muscle groups that you want to emphasize.

Mistake # 3: Misuse of dirty meals

Most fitness enthusiasts think they need dirty meals too often.

Once because of a heavy workout, once because the diet was missed, once again because a holiday is coming, and so on.

Frequent dirty meals can have a negative effect not only by drastically increasing calorie intake but also on inflammatory processes.

Perhaps it has happened to you after a big pizza to feel stomach discomfort for hours, something that rarely happens when you eat healthy food.

This negative is not just momentary. There is also the potential to prevent the absorption of nutrients for several days ahead, which in turn seriously damages your progress.

Mistake # 4: Alcohol and dirty meals

Alcohol cannot be stored as subcutaneous fat.

The problem of alcohol consumption is that it gives extra calories and at the same time it blocks the oxidation of fat in a similar way to carbohydrates.

The result of this process is less of a body's ability to use fat for energy because it first has to "burn" alcohol.

So alcohol consumption in moderate amounts would not do much harm, but regular consumption will not allow the body to use accumulated fat as a source of energy.

Here are some basic tips to help reduce alcohol-related harm:

• Do not consume more than 1-2 times a week;

• Reduce fat intake the same day;

• Do not eat high fat foods along with alcohol consumption;

• Avoid drinks that contain added carbohydrates and sugar - beer, cocktails.

How can dirty meals benefit then?

For each potential negative there is also a corresponding positive that can be extracted.

Benefit # 1: Mental Retirement

In case you are rational in your choices, you can use dirty meals for mental relaxation.

Knowing that you deserved a Saturday meal with friends outside can be a prerequisite for working harder throughout the week.

Benefit # 2: Hormonal Benefits

When a certain point in fat loss is reached, consumption of high calorie feed can stimulate the process (fat burning) for the next few days.

With a drastic reduction in subcutaneous fat or tight diets, the thyroid function decreases significantly and leptin levels respectively.

A bigger flow of calories can work positively in this case as long as it's done properly - without overeating.

Benefit # 3: Filling of glycogen

If you feel tired and feel your body flat, dirty food can fill your muscles with glycogen again when you really need it.

Benefit # 4: Balanced Tool

Dirty food can be used as a tool for balancing physics.

For example, if biceps and triceps are a weak muscle group, a dirty diet around hand training can positively affect giving more energy, protecting the muscles and feeding more nutrients than usual.

How to enjoy dirty meals without derailing your regime?

• Make a plan and have an idea when it will take place;

• Use dirty meals to get extra benefits;

• Preferably choose foods that are not only calorie but also nutritional;

• Do not consume alcohol in combination with high calorie foods (especially fat sources);

• If you want to make a big dirty meal, remove some of the calories from previous meals.

In Conclusion

According to my observations, many fitness enthusiasts try to justify their bad choices with dirty meals without first having put themselves in a position where they can benefit from them.

For example, if you feel that you need to disrupt your regime every 4-5 days, you are likely not to make much progress with your fitness goals, so think about what needs to be done in your plan.

On the other hand, if you can use methodically and logically dirty meals as a plus, you do not need to feel guilty.

Also, remember that it matters what dirty food you choose.

Dirty home-cooked meals can be much better controlled by calories than dirty meals from a restaurant where there are often additional hidden calories from sources such as butter and sugar.

And once again: dirty food is just 1 meal, not food consumption, which is supposed to not be consumed throughout the day.

If you follow the 90/10 rule, you have a greater chance of keeping a diet or diet easier in the long run, and those 10% will not prevent you from losing weight, shaping the desired body or keeping results.

I am introducing you three diets: Balanced Diet, Vegetarian Diet and Vegan Diet for those who like these types of eating

9 DAYS NORMAL DIET

DAY 1 AND 2

1.Breakfast at 8 AM

Always optional coffee or tea with or without milk.

Fresh vegetables - carrots or fruit juice.

Option 1

     150-200 grams of vegetables - cucumbers and carrots / parsley and carrot juice + 2 boiled eggs.

Option 2

    A cup of almond or coconut bio-milk without sugar / or yogurt 150-200 ml + 3-4 tablespoons pre-soaked oatmeal mixture, ground sesame and pumpkin seeds, almonds.

2.One hour before lunch

Vegetable cuttings + mozzarella or cottage cheese 50-60 g

or

Vegetable or fruit smoothie 250-300 ml

3.Lunch at 1-2 PM

Salad of your choice 200-250g with 1-2 tsp. olive oil, a little balsamic vinegar or lemon, moderate salt:

- cucumber, iceberg, cherry, carrot, baby spinach, avocado - optional

- Optional fruit 250-300 g

+

- Portion a second dish or soup 250-300g

or

- stewed green beans with vegetables, mushrooms

or

- a cup of yoghurt

or

- cream soup of broccoli / vegetables + mozzarella 50-60 g or other cheese

or

- spinach with egg

4.Afternoon at 5 PM.

200-250 ml fresh vegetables - carrots for example + 10-12 hazelnuts

or

- a portion of yoghurt 200-250 ml

or

- Vegetable with nuts

or

- Vegetable cuttings + 1 boiled egg

5.Dinner at 8 PM.

- portion salad vegetables optional 200-250 g with 1-2 tsp. olive oil, lemon, or balsamic, moderate salt

+ meal / soup 250-300 ml from lunchtime meal

or

 salad + fish / seafood 200-250g

DAY 3 AND 4

1.Breakfast at 8 AM

Option 1

1.2-3 cuttings ready fish fillet 40-50 r

Or

2-3 cuttings of ham

+

2. Vegetables - cucumber / 1-2 sheets of iceberg / cherry or pepper

+

3. Boiled egg

 At breakfast you can consume different options, for example:

 1 + 2 + 3 or 1+ 2 or 3 + 1, etc.

Option 2

Cucumber and carrot cuttings + omelet - 2 eggs + 50g ham

2.One hour before lunch

Fresh vegetables 250-300 ml

3.Lunch at 1-2 PM

1. Salad 200-250 g with 1-2 tsp. olive oil or oil / linseed oil or oil grape seed, moderate salt, lemon or apple vinegar

   - cucumbers / green salad / iceberg / peppers / carrots / cabbage / icebergs / etc. optionally

2. A second dish or soup 250-300 g:

- Fish 200-250 g / seafood 200 g + Vegetables per pan

- steak + vegetable puree without potatoes and no milk

- zucchini stuffed with lean minced meat and vegetables

- meat / bird in oven with zucchini, peppers, mushrooms

- Chicken soup

4.Afternoon at 4-5 PM

cucumber / raw pepper + 2-3 slices of fish fillet /

or

 tuna can with vegetables

or

2-3 pieces of turkey or chicken ham 40-50g

or

- green salad - iceberg, tuna cucumber and boiled egg

5.Dinner at 8 PM

1.One salad of your choice 200-250 g with olive oil, apple vinegar, moderate salt

+

2. Portion of lunch meals and soup 250-300 g

DAY 5 AND 6

1.Breakfast at 8 AM

OPTION 1:

1. raw red pepper / carrot

2. 50 g mozzarella / fresh cheese - cottage cheese -1-2 tsp.

3.fresh olives 7-8 pcs.

4.Sugar-free jam

+ a slice of whole grain bread

Option 2:

pre-soaked Grain mixture - oat bran, ground linseed and raw seeds of pumpkin or sunflower - a total of 3-4 tablespoons that mix with a glass of yoghurt or coconut, almond milk

Option 3:

Omelet with cheese + vegetable cuttings

2.One hour before lunch

300gr. Fruits

- or a glass of yoghurt + 2-3 tsp. soaked oat bran and chia OR + raspberries or blueberries

- chocolate without sugar

or

Chocolate mousse or ice cream without sugar with nuts and fruits

3.Lunch at 1-2 PM

 Salad 200-250 g with 1-2 tsp. olive oil and some salt, lemon

1. Second dish / soup 300 ml:

or

- vegetables baked in an oven with yoghurt and egg

or

peas with vegetables

or

- brown rice with vegetables

or

- Spaghetti with cheese or with vegetables

or

sweet potatoes with vegetables

4.Afternoon at 4-5 PM

- vegetables + 50-60 g + boiled egg

or

- Stuffed pepper with cottage cheese / ricotta /

or

- Fresh - chopped vegetables + raw nuts or seeds

5.Dinner at 8 PM

OPTION 1

1.Salad 250-300 g with 1 tsp. olive oil and vinegar and salt moderately

2.Portion 250-300 ml of second meal or soup lunch menu without dairy products or

- seafood + vegetables on pan-grill

- baked fish 250 g + steamed vegetables

OPTION 2

A large portion of salad 400-500 g of iceberg, green salad, cucumber with 2 tablespoons tuna and boiled egg.

DAY 7

1.Breakfast

- carrots and cucumber slices / fresh carrots 300 ml

+2 boiled eggs

Or vegetable soup 300 ml + 2 tablespoons oat bran + cucumber slices

2. Before lunch and before dinner

Vegetables / fresh vegetables 200 ml + 10-12 raw nuts

or

- vegetable smoothie

or

- fresh fruit 200-250 ml

or

- or 300 ml of low-fat yoghurt

3.Lunch and Dinner

- salad vegetables 200-250 g with olive oil 1 tsp, lemon or vinegar, moderate salt

+ 250 ml soup vegetables / or + vegetables on pan without potatoes 300 g

Or + zucchini, peppers / or stewed green beans 250 g

Or dinner 200 g of seafood + stewed asparagus / broccoli / cauliflower

DAY 8 AND 9

1.Breakfast

Option 1

1.1-2 pcs. Boiled eggs

2. Vegetables

3. Two pieces turkey ham or fillet

4. Fish fillet + vegetables

Option 2

Omelet 2 eggs, ham 50 g + vegetable cuttings

2.Lunch

Salad normal portion 250-300 g with 1 tsp. olive oil, salt, lemon or vinegar

- salad cucumber with dill

- green salad with or without cucumbers

- salad iceberg, baby spinach, cucumber, avokado

- Peeled tomatoes and cucumbers

- Roasted peppers with parsley and dill

- Zucchini salad

2. Second optional dish:

Stewed green beans

- Bird or meat with spinach

- Turkey / lean meat with vegetables without potatoes

- Veal boiled without potatoes, but with other vegetables

- Of course, always a portion of baked fish + vegetables on a pan / grill / without potatoes

- Omelet with 2 eggs and ham

- Rabbit with vegetables

3.Afternoon at 4-5 PM

Fillet of choice / ham light 2-3 cuttings / fish fillet + vegetables of choice

- Tomato juice / carrot juice without sugar + sliced two ham or turkey fillet

4.Dinner

1.Salad 200-250 g with olive oil, moderate salt and lemon or vinegar

- cucumbers and tomatoes

- Salad cucumbers and dill or

- Iceberg with cucumbers

+

- 2. Second dish from the lunch menu optional 250-300g

ENJOY

9 DAYS VEGETARIAN DIET

1 AND 2 DAYS

1.Breakfast

1-2 eggs

2-3 tablespoons cheese

1-2 pcs. tomatoes

Roasted / raw red peppers 3-4 pcs.

10-12 medium-sized, very well desalted black olives

2.Around 11 AM. - 300 g of fruit - 1-2 grapefruit, 2-3 apples, pomegranate, roasted pumpkin without honey and sugar, but can be sprinkled with ground walnuts.

3.Lunch

1. Salad 250-300 g with 1-2 tsp. olive oil, lemon / balsamic vinegar and a little potassium salt to taste but without cheese.

- Salad tomatoes and cucumbers, onion or

- Salad roasted or roasted peppers with tomatoes or,

- Cucumber salad or,

- Green salad with cucumbers, fresh onions and optionally broccoli and seeds.

2.Second meal of the following vegetables:

- Fresh zucchini

- Peeled tomatoes

- Green beans

- Cleaned and cut mushrooms

- Desalted black olives

- For flavor use onions, fresh garlic, lots of parsley + savory + oregano + little salt / + 3-4 tsp. vegetable oil.

/ Zucchini + sliced peppers, tomato onions and onions, mushrooms, savory and parsley baked in an oven /

or

/ Vegetables on grill pan or grill from the listed /

or

/ mushrooms with vegetables /

With regard to the quantity and proportion of the ingredients of the above vegetables you have no limitation, it is not necessary to use all the vegetables.

4.Around 4 PM.

Vegetable salad with 1-2 tsp. olive oil in one serving

/ If you are still hungry 20-30 minutes after the salad, a 250-300g portion of the lunch meal /

5. Dinner around 7 PM.

1. Salad - tomatoes, cucumbers and peppers up to 250-300g

or

/ salad cucumbers with more dill and parsley, roasted peppers with garlic and parsley / with 1 tbsp. olive oil + a little salt

2. Vegetables in oven 1 portion 300 g / peppers, mushrooms, tomatoes, onion on oven.

or

Vegetables on grill pan.

DAY 3 AND 4

1.Breakfast

Desalted green olives 12-15 pcs.

Roasted / raw / green peppers 4-5 pcs.

Half cucumber /

Soy cheese - tofu 50-60 g

2.Around 11 AM.

2-3 kiwi

/ a few pre-soaked prunes or apples or oranges and drink the water in which they are sipped.

3.Lunch around 1 – 2 PM.

1. Salad 1 serving 250-300 g

- Salad tomatoes and cucumbers / tomatoes with roasted peppers, cucumbers, green salad / 1-2 tsp. olive oil and very little potassium salt

/ maybe two types of salads, again respecting the quantity /

2.Soup of vegetables not stuffed / stewed or steamed vegetables / of the following vegetables:

- Cauliflower

- White cabbage to 2-3 cups pre-cut

- Carrots 2-3 pieces for the whole dish

- Tomatoes peeled

- Mushrooms cut into strips

- 1-2 potatoes pre-peeled

- onion

- dill, parsley to your taste + a little salt / + 2-3 tsp. vegetable oil /

Depending on your preference, you may not add all the ingredients to the soup again.

4.Around 4 PM.

Salad 250-300 g of choice from the recommended + 1-2 tablespoons nuts raw almonds.

5.Dinner around 7-8 PM.

1.Salad with desalinated olives 300-400 g with 1-2 tsp. olive oil, a little potassium salt and lemon.

/ Green salad, salad tomatoes and cucumbers up to 350-400 g, salad only from cucumbers and green desalinated olives, salad carrots, turnip and olives /

2. Portion-two soup from vegetables 300 g /

Or

Peppers, carrots, mushrooms and tomatoes in oven /

DAY 5

1.Breakfast

Cucumber 1-2 pcs.

Roasted peppers 2-3 pcs.

Desalted Olives 8-10 pcs.

Bread 1-2 slices

2.Around 11 AM.

Baked fruits - apples, quince, pumpkin, kiwi - about 300-400 g + 1-2 tablespoons raw pumpkin seeds or sunflower seeds.

3.Lunch

1.Salad - tomatoes, cucumbers and red peppers up to 400-500 g (2 servings) with 2 tsp. olive oil and a little salt to taste, lemon.

or

/ Salad carrots, desalted black olives and 1 tablespoon. raw sunflower seeds peeled /

or

/ Salad green, onion, cucumbers and radish + green olives /

or

/ Only salad cucumbers with more dill and parsley /

4.Around 4-5 PM.

Salad or 300 g of fruit accepted before lunch

5.Dinner

500 g salad only cucumbers

Or

/ Tomatoes + peppers + cucumbers + fresh onions / 1-2 tsp. olive oil and some salt, lemon according to your wishes.

or

/ Green salad with cucumber, green onion and broccoli, seeds, soy, etc. /

There are no restrictions on the quantity of salad accepted and for lunch and dinner.

It can be increased if necessary and feeling hungry.

If this feeling is strong take a portion of the soup / lunch meal / from the previous day or prepare a new quantity.

DAY 6

Repeat day 5!

DAY 7

Repeat day 3!

DAY 8

Repeat the 1st day, adding to 1-2 boiled eggs for breakfast and dinner.

DAY 9

1.Breakfast

2-3 tablespoons cottage cheese + 1-2 boiled eggs

10-12 desalted black olives

2-3 roasted or raw peppers

Half cucumber

2. Around 11 AM.

2-3 kiwi, baked fruit, bowl 250-300 g raspberries, 2 apples it is up to you.

3.Lunch

1. Salad 250-300 gr. with 1-2 tsp. olive oil and a little salt, lemon

- Cucumbers + Parsley

or

- Green salad with cucumbers, radishes, onions

2.Soup of vegetables - a portion of about 250-300 ml. on the recipe of the 3rd day

3. One dish

/ zucchini in oven + peppers + mushrooms + onion + dill /

4.Around 4-5 PM.

A portion of 250-300 g of the soup or salad 1 serving

Or

/ whole vegetables + 1-2 tablespoons raw sunflower or pumpkin seeds /

5.Dinner

1.Salad tomatoes, cucumbers and peppers 250-300 g with 1-2 tsp. olive oil + a little salt and lemon

or

/ Cucumbers with green salad, radishes, olives and 1 - 2 pcs. eggs /

2.White fish fillet cooked on steam - about 150 g /

Or

Boiled chicken fillet without skin 100 g / + vegetables broccoli, cauliflower, steamed peppers, grill or steamed.

During the entire period of this regime:

1. Drink enough water even if you do not feel thirsty up to 2 liters daily only water - mineral, table, boiled or green or herbal tea.

Immediately after getting up / cup-two slightly warm up before sleeping on a glass of water.

2. If you feel weakness or dizziness add additional food that is planned for the day.

It will not be fatal if you eat more than planned vegetables, salads and dishes.

Avoid fruits in the evening after a meal.

For breakfast and lunch, we accept 1-2 slices bread.

If you feel weakness drink a cup of tea with 1 tsp. honey !

Except for fruits and bread, you can improvise within the recommended product range of the day, but it is advisable to start avoiding food intake after 10 PM in the evening.

ENJOY!!!

9-DAY VEGAN DIET

DAY 1 AND 2

1. Breakfast

Option 1

150-200 g of vegetables - cucumbers and carrots / carrot juice 250 ml + 12-15 raw almond / hazelnut

Option 2

Cup of coconut, almond or soy milk 200 ml + 3-4 tablespoons the pre-soaked mixture of oat bran, chia, sesame and pumpkin seeds and ½ tsp. cinnamon

2. Before Lunch

Option 1

- 15-18 raw almonds

Option 2

- Vegetable smoothie with 1 tablespoon chia, 1 tablespoon bran several raw almonds - 200 ml

Option 3

- Fresh carrots 200-250 ml / carrots and cucumber slices + 10-12 raw nuts

3. Lunch

Option 1

-Salad (your choice) 200-250g with 1-2 tsp. olive oil, a little vinegar or lemon, moderate salt:

Option 2

- Cucumber, iceberg, carrots, anchovies, baby spinach - optional

+

-. Portion of second dish or soup 250-300g

- Stewed green beans with dill

- Steamed spinach

4. Afternoon 4-5 PM.

Option 1

- 200-250 ml fresh of vegetables - carrots with or without 10-12 almonds

Option 2

- vegetable smoothie with 250 ml nuts

Option 3

- vegetable cuttings carrots, peppers, cucumbers 200 g

5. Dinner

- Salad - cucumber, pepper 200-250 g with 1-2 tsp. olive oil, lemon, moderate salt

+

Meal 250-300g left from the lunch

DAY 3 AND 4

1. Breakfast

Option 1

Vegetable Cream Soup without potatoes 250 ml + cucumber cuttings 100 g

Option 2

- Cucumbers and carrots + tofu 50-60 g

Option 3

- Mixture of ground flaxseed, oatmeal, raw sunflower seeds, dried fruit - raisins, apricots, almonds or hazelnuts

2. Before Lunch

Option 1

Fruits 250-300g optional without bananas and grapes

Option 2

Fruit juice 200 ml + several raw nuts or 1-2 tablespoons raw peeled sunflower seeds

Option 3

3-4 walnuts

3.Lunch

- Salad 250 300g with addition of 1-2 olive oil and a little salt

or

- Salad cucumbers + iceberg and spring onion

or

- Peppers and cucumbers, avocados

or

- Salad cucumbers with dill, peppers

or

- Salad carrots with olives

+

Second choice of meal 250-300 g:

-Cream soup of Broccoli + tofu 30-40 g

- Roasted pepper, zucchini, carrots, mushrooms

4. Before Dinner 4-5 PM.

Optional

- 2-3 walnuts

- Avocado + nuts and seeds - 150 g

5. Dinner

- Repeat lunch options:

- Salad 250-300 g with 1 tsp. olive oil, salt

+

- Second dish or soup 250-300 ml.

DAY 5 AND 6

1. Breakfast

Option 1

150-200 g of vegetables - cucumbers and carrots / carrot juice 250 ml + 12-15 raw almond / hazelnut

Option 2

Cup of coconut, almond or soy milk 200 ml + 3-4 tablespoons pre-soaked mixture of oat bran, chia and pumpkin seeds and ½ tsp. cinnamon

2. Before Lunch

- 15-18 raw almonds

- Vegetable smoothie with 1 tablespoon chia, 1 tablespoon bran several raw almonds - 200 ml

- Fresh of carrots 200-250 ml

3. Lunch

Option 1

-Salad (your choice) 200-250g with 1-2 tsp. olive oil, a little vinegar or lemon, moderate salt:

Option 2

- Cucumber, iceberg, carrots, anchovies, baby spinach - optional

+

-. Portion of second dish or soup 250-300g

- Stewed green beans with dill

- Steamed spinach

4. Afternoon 4-5 PM.

Option 1

- 200-250 ml fresh of vegetables - carrots with or without 10-12 almonds

Option 2

- Vegetable smoothie with 250 ml nuts

Option 3

- Vegetable cuttings carrots, peppers, cucumbers 200 g

5. Dinner

- Salad - cucumber, pepper 200-250 g with 1-2 tsp. olive oil, lemon, moderate salt

+

Meal 250-300g left from the lunch

DAY 7 AND 8

1. Breakfast

Option 1

Fresh vegetables - carrots for example 250 ml + 12-15 raw nuts pre-soaked in water

Option 2

  Soy milk 1 cup 200 ml + 3-4 tablespoons pre-soaked oatmeal mixture, oat bran and nuts

Option 3

  Humus 100-150 gr.

2. Before Lunch

Option 1

- Optional fruit 250-300 g without bananas and grapes - mango, papaya, blueberries, strawberries

Option 2

- Vegetable smoothie of green vegetables and apple + 1-2 tablespoon of raw seeds and nuts

3. Lunch

- Salad by your choice 250-300 gr. with olive oil, salt and lemon

+

Cream soup with 2 tbs. oat bran or chia

or

Tomatoes cream soup

or

- To the salad only 40-50 gr. tofu

4. Afternoon (4-5 PM.)

Option 1

- 200-250 ml fresh of vegetables - carrots with or without 10-12 almonds

Option 2

- Vegetable smoothie with 250 ml nuts

Option 3

- Vegetable cuttings carrots, peppers, cucumbers 200 g

5. Dinner

- Salad 250-300 g with 1 tsp. olive oil, salt

+

- Second dish or soup 250-300 ml.

DAY 9

1.Breakfast

2 sliced whole-grain bread desalted

+ tofu cheese 30-40 g + vegetable cuttings

+ 5-6 olives

2.Before lunch

Option 1

- Vegan chocolate without sugar 40-50g

or cereal protein bar 1 pc.

Option 2

- vegan cream with coconut

- Whole-grain pancake with sugar-free jam

3.Lunch

-Salad 200-250g with 1-2 tsp. olive oil, a little vinegar or lemon, moderate salt:

- Green, cucumber, iceberg, carrots, anchovies, baby spinach - optional

-

+

-. Portion a second dish or soup 250-300g

- Potato oven vegetables

- Whole grain spaghetti with vegetables and mushrooms or with cashew cheese

- Vegetables with brown rice / cinnamon - - Zucchini, peppers, carrots, cauliflower, mushrooms

- Vegetables baked with tomato sauce

- Broccoli and cauliflower baked in an oven with shredded tofu

- Beans with vegetables

- Lentil soup

- Vegan sushi

4.Before dinner 4-5 PM.

- 200-250 ml fresh vegetables - carrots for example + 12-15 raw hazelnuts

or

- Vegetable smoothie with nuts

or

- Vegetable cuttings + 15-20 tofu, nuts

- Cream soup vegetables + 1-2 tablespoons chia or oat bran

5.Dinner

- a portion of salad 200-250g

+ Main dish / soup 250-300 ml but without potatoes, spaghetti and rice!

For example baked peppers, zucchini, egplant with tomato sauce.

ENJOY!

In short, optimal nutrition includes an adequate product set, good diet, good food preparation, water intake. It is difficult to escape the tension, and the air is as we have it. When we can get out of the mountains from time to time, and tension can be fought with a good motor activity. Positive mood is also very important - to smile more, to believe more, to be less frightened, more critical of ourselves and less to others. If we are more critical of ourselves, perhaps we will be better off. This is more important.

When we are healthy, we can be more useful to others, to the closest people. This is in two words. The latter is my creed.

One should not be given both drastic excesses and deprivation. Let's have the little sweet things in life - like food too. We have to respect what will be pleasant and having a good eating system, we can make small deviations, as long as they remain small deviations, not the rule.

Eat to be healthy. Feeding is good to be alkaline, to help hepatic function, the function of our excretory system to promote good water balance, and the result will always be in the face. The body is a system, through nutrition we must create the necessary conditions for this system to work. It can self-regulate. And despite heredity, be on a good level.

One should take care of their own health, not just wait for help from outside. He must first take good care of himself by doing all that is necessary to establish his condition. Especially if there is a complaint. Then, knowing his condition, turning to a specialist and getting the right information, must be able to apply it. If he is interested in himself until symptoms occur, it may be too late. When a person has a good, balanced diet that is in tune and is adequate to his or her health problems, it would put them under control or delay their negative effect over time. If he is healthy, it would be a prerequisite for many years to flee from, and not against, different health issues. Accepting adequate food and water, breathing fresh air, motor activity helps all of these factors affect it with minimal damaging effects.

The more people have overweight and obesity, the more society starts to consider it normal. As a result, people who suffer from this problem are becoming more prone to not take action to deal with it, but only to look for temporary solutions for instant weight loss. This is a serious problem because overweight and obesity are not just aesthetic problems.

The health risks of overweight and especially obesity are many. Some include:

• Cardiac and cerebrovascular diseases, including heart attack and stroke

• Increased insulin resistance and diabetes